Selected Bibliography of Pediatric Orthopaedics With Commentary

Edited by
Walter B. Greene, MD
Professor of Orthopaedic Surgery and Pediatrics
Division of Orthopaedics
The University of North Carolina School of Medicine
Chapel Hill, North Carolina

Eric T. Jones, MD
Clinical Professor of Pediatric Orthopaedic Surgery
West Virginia University
Morgantown, West Virginia

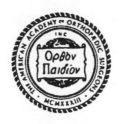

American Academy of Orthopaedic Surgeons
222 S. Prospect Avenue
Park Ridge, Illinois 60068

International Standard Book Number: 0-89203-038-0
Library of Congress Catalog Card Number: 90-62232

Table of Contents

Preface

The third edition of the *Selected Bibliography of Pediatric Orthopaedics With Commentary* continues the efforts initiated in 1970 when the American Academy of Orthopaedic Surgeons published a *Study Guide in Pediatric Orthopaedics*. The reference was prepared by the Academy's Committee for the Care of the Handicapped Child. The first edition of the *Selected Bibliography of Pediatric Orthopaedics* was published in 1980 and the second in 1985. These editions, like the present one, were prepared by the Committee on Pediatric Orthopaedics. Prefaces to previous editions have recognized individuals who were instrumental in initiating and organizing this bibliography. We would only add that the work of Brian L. Hotchkiss, MD, editor of the second edition, was paramount in producing that volume in a timely fashion.

The third edition reviews publications through 1989. The listing of articles is not intended to be exhaustive. The intent has been to publish a reasonable bibliographic overview of the subject to serve as a departure point for those interested in further study.

The authors listed for each section reviewed previous editions, searched the literature for the intervening years, selected the appropriate articles to include in this bibliography, and wrote the annotations. Much of the credit for this resource goes to these individuals and to the contributors of previous editions whose selections and a notations are still being used.

The publications staff of the Academy is to be commended for another expeditious and capable job. In particular we would like to acknowledge the efforts of Bruce A. Davis, who managed the editorial process; Monica M. Trocker, who directed word processing efforts; Marilyn L. Fox, PhD, who provided overall direction for the publication; and Mark W. Wieting, who is director of the Academy's Department of Communications and Publications. Lastly, the Board of Directors of the Academy are to be commended for their support in this and many other functions that augment our continued education in orthopaedic surgery and the resultant improvement in patient care.

Walter B. Greene, MD

Eric T. Jones, MD

History of Orthopaedics

Vernon Tolo, MD

Fifty years of orthopaedics. Ponseti IV. *J Pediatr Orthop* 1989;9:79-85.
As the guest lecturer at the 1988 American Academy of Orthopaedic Surgeons annual meeting, Dr. Ponseti traces the transformation of "orthopaedics from a specialty with much empirical craftsmanship into an important scientific discipline." In a well-articulated presentation, he relates the basic science discoveries over this time to changes in orthopaedic care, particularly related to children.

Anthology of Orthopaedics. Rang M. Edinburgh, E & S Livingstone, 1966.
Though not new, this book remains a major source for biographical information about early orthopaedists whose names are now used as eponyms.

Fifty Years of Progress. Heck CV. Chicago, American Academy of Orthopaedic Surgeons, 1983.
Written on the occasion of the 50th anniversary of the American Academy of Orthopaedic Surgeons, this book traces the evolution of the Academy.

Source Book of Orthopaedics. Bick EM. New York, Hafner, 1968.
Extensive reference source for early orthopaedic writing.

The Early Orthopaedic Surgeons of America. Shands AR Jr. St. Louis, CV Mosby, 1970.

Selected Classics (as reprinted in *Clinical Orthopaedics and Related Research*)
The classic: Contributions to the radical treatment of congenital unilateral coxo-femoral dislocation. Poggi A. *Clin Orthop* 1974;98:5-7.
First major paper to include acetabular surgery as a part of operative treatment for congenital hip dislocation.

The classic: Kyphosis dorsalis juvenilis. Scheuermann HW. *Clin Orthop* 1977;128:5-7.
Initial report of the spinal deformity that bears the author's name.

The classic: Deformities of the human frame. Little WJ. *Clin Orthop* 1978;131:3-9.
The first clear description of cerebral palsy in children.

The classic: Growth and predictions of growth in the lower extremities. Anderson M, Green WT, Messner MB. *Clin Orthop* 1978;136:7-21. (Reprinted from Messner AB. *J Bone Joint Surg* 1963;45A:1.)
> Reports the development of growth curves based on a study of growth in 50 boys and 50 girls measured at least once a year over their last eight years of growth.

The classic: On a particular form of pseudo-coxalgia associated with a characteristic deformity of the upper end of the femur. Calvé J. *Clin Orthop* 1980;150:4-7.
> The initial French report of a childhood hip disorder now known to be due to avascular necrosis but previously thought to be caused by tuberculosis.

The classic: Concerning arthritis deformans juvenilis. Perthes GC; Peltier LF, trans-ed. *Clin Orthop* 1981;158:5-9.
> The initial German report of the childhood hip condition now known by the author's name.

The classic: A typical disease of the upper femoral epiphysis. Schwarz E. *Clin Orthop* 1986;209:5-12.
> An early description of the avascular etiology of Legg-Calvé-Perthes disease in childhood.

The classic: Support for the spondylitic spine by means of buried steel bars, attached to the vertebrae. Lange F. *Clin Orthop* 1986;203:3-6.
> A report from 1910 describing the use of metallic implants for internal fixation of the spine.

The classic: A human monster with inwardly curved extremities. Otto AW. *Clin Orthop* 1985;194:4-5.
> The first clinical description of a child with arthrogryposis multiplex congenita.

The classic: Separations of the epiphyses. Foucher JTE; Peltier LF, trans-ed. *Clin Orthop* 1984;188:3-9.
> Published in 1867, this paper describes clinical and cadaver studies of how and when physeal disruptions occur.

Concerning the interrelationship between form and function of the individual parts of the organism. Wolff J. *Clin Orthop* 1988;228:2-11.
> This paper from 1900 describes "Wolff's law."

A report of fifty-nine cases of scoliosis treated by the fusion operation. Hibbs RA. *Clin Orthop* 1988;229:4-19.
> The first significant series reported on the surgical treatment of scoliosis by spinal fusion. (Reprinted from *J Bone Joint Surg* 1924;6:3.)

Preface to "A treatise on the nature of club-foot and analogous distortions; including their treatment both with and without surgical operation. Illustrated by a series of cases and numerous practical instructions." Little WJ. *Clin Orthop* 1988;233:3-6.

> A description from 1839 of Little's experience in England with heelcord lengthening (an operation Stromeyer had performed on Little himself in 1835 in Germany) for a variety of equinus conditions.

Growth and Development of the Musculoskeletal System

David P. Roye Jr, MD

The Musculoskeletal System: Basic Processes and Disorders, ed 2. Wilson FC (ed). Philadelphia, JB Lippincott, 1983.
> This textbook presents easy-to-understand concepts of growth and development. It is written primarily for the medical student.

Development and maturation of the neuromusculoskeletal system. Ogden JA. In Morrissy RT (ed): *Lovell and Winter's Pediatric Orthopaedics*, ed 3. Philadelphia, JB Lippincott, 1990.
> This well-stated chapter covers the development of the spinal cord and vertebra as well as the mechanisms of long-bone growth.

Bone Diseases of Children. Maroteaux P. Philadelphia, JB Lippincott, 1979.
> This text provides essential information on normal growth and development, followed by an in-depth presentation of skeletal disorders of growth.

Developmental pediatrics: Growth and development. Vaughan VC III. In Behrman RE, Vaughan VC III (eds): *Nelson Textbook of Pediatrics,* ed 13. Philadelphia, WB Saunders, 1987, chap 2, pp 6-112.
> Pediatric growth and development relating to the whole child including the musculoskeletal system.

Basic Science

Anatomy and physiology of skeletal development. Ogden JA. *Skeletal Injury in the Child.* Philadelphia, Lea & Febiger, 1982, chap 2, pp 16-40.
> This chapter emphasizes the effects of injury to various regions of the skeletal system.

Embryology and spine growth. Lonstein JE. In Bradford DS, Lonstein JE, Moe JH, et al (eds): *Moe's Textbook of Scoliosis and Other Spinal Deformities*, ed 2. Philadelphia, WB Saunders, 1987, chap 3, pp 25-40.

Bone Circulation. Arlet J, Ficat RP, Hungerford DS (eds). Baltimore, Williams & Wilkins, 1984.
> Excellent basic science data on bone circulation and how it affects growth of bone. Contains multiple short chapters on limited subjects.

The uniqueness of growing bones. Ogden JA. In Rockwood CA Jr, Wilkins KE, King RE (eds): *Fractures in Children*. Philadelphia, JB Lippincott, 1984, vol 3, chap 1, pp 1-86.
> This chapter on bone growth distills much that is in the literature. A "must-read" for orthopaedic residents.

Growth and early development of the musculoskeletal system. Hensinger RN, Jones ET. *Neonatal Orthopaedics*. New York, Grune & Stratton, 1981, chap 2, pp 5-13.
> This chapter discusses early development in the neonatal period.

Studies of the Development and Decay of the Human Frame. Trueta J. Philadelphia, WB Saunders, 1968.
> One of the best collections of original research in this field, this book contains many "pearls" about anatomy and physiology of the musculoskeletal system. Out of print, but available in many libraries.

Clinical Conditions

Gait Disorders in Childhood and Adolescence. Sutherland DH. Baltimore, Williams & Wilkins, 1984.
> A good discussion of lower extremity patterns of development with special emphasis on how gait is affected.

Limb Development and Deformity: Problems of Evaluation and Rehabilitation. Swinyard CA (ed). Springfield, IL, Charles C Thomas, 1969.
> A classic. Somewhat outdated, but still an excellent resource text with many fine illustrations.

Regression of femoral anteversion: A prospective study of intoeing children. Svenningsen S, Apalset K, Terjesen T, et al. *Acta Orthop Scand* 1989;60:170-173.
> This well documented study covers the natural history of femoral neck anteversion and is a nice addition to classic studies.

Growth and predictions of growth in the upper extremity. Pritchett JW. *J Bone Joint Surg* 1988;70A:520-525.
> In this excellent reference for predicting upper extremity growth patterns 244 children were followed to maturity.

Angular deformities of the lower limbs in children. Kling TF Jr. *Orthop Clin North Am* 1987;18:513-527.
> This excellent review of congenital deformities includes the natural history of physiologic varus and valgus and refers to many worthwhile articles on pediatric lower extremity problems.

Longitudinal bone growth: The growth plate and its dysfunctions. Brighton CT. In Griffin PP (ed): American Academy of Orthopaedic Surgeons

Instructional Course Lectures, XXXVI. Park Ridge, IL, American Academy of Orthopaedic Surgeons, 1987, pp 3-25.
> This excellent review of growth plate functions provides good insight into normal and abnormal functioning of the growth plate.

Lower-extremity rotational problems in children: Normal values to guide management. Staheli LT, Corbett M, Wyss C, et al. *J Bone Joint Surg* 1985;67A:39-47.
> A natural history study, this paper documents normal variations and changes associated with growth. Essential information.

Origin and mechanism of postnatal deformities. Bunch W. *Pediatr Clin North Am* 1977;24:679-684.
> A fine discussion of this topic aimed at the pediatrician. This issue also has other good chapters which apply to this area.

The development of mature gait. Sutherland DH, Olshen R, Cooper L, et al. *J Bone Joint Surg* 1980;62A:336-353.
> Detailed gait studies were performed and analyzed on 186 normal children between the ages of 1 and 7 years. Sagittal-plane angular motion is similar to that in normal adults by age 2 years. Reciprocal arm swing and heel strike are present by 18 months. Step length and walking velocity increase with growth while cadence decreases. Only minor differences in gait are seen in a 7-year-old compared with an adult.

Genetics and Syndromes

Michael J. Goldberg, MD

The Dysmorphic Child: An Orthopedic Perspective. Goldberg MJ. New York, Raven Press, 1987.
> Presents the musculoskeletal and significant nonorthopaedic aspects of the most frequently encountered syndromes. Emphasizes the differential diagnosis of children with similar extremity and spine deformities.

Mendelian Inheritance in Man: Catalogs of Autosomal Dominant, Autosomal Recessive, and X-linked Phenotypes, ed 8. McKusick VA. Baltimore, Johns Hopkins University Press, 1988.
> An encyclopedic listing of genetically transmitted disorders. Also includes essential basic clinical information, detailed biochemistry, and an up-to-date bibliography.

Smith's Recognizable Patterns of Human Malformation, ed 4. Smith DW, Jones KL. Philadelphia, WB Saunders, 1988.
> Previous editions of Smith's textbook established it as the standard of a beautifully illustrated and concise textbook of dysmorphology. This edition by Jones continues the tradition.

Clinical Atlas of Human Chromosomes, ed 2. de Grouchy J, Turleau C. New York, John Wiley & Sons, 1984.
> In a rapidly changing field, this remains a well illustrated guide to the chromosomal syndromes.

The Genetics of Hand Malformations. Temtamy SA, McKusick VA. New York, AR Liss, 1978.
> Still the definitive work on upper extremity malformations of every type.

Principles and Practice of Medical Genetics. Emery AEH, Rimoin DL (eds). Edinburgh, Churchill Livingstone, 1983.
> This comprehensive work has detailed chapters on almost every genetic disorder but has become a bit out of date.

Medical Genetics: Principles and Practice, ed 3. Nora JJ, Fraser FC. Philadelphia, Lea & Febiger, 1989.
> This soft-bound book, an excellent introduction to human genetics, includes both basic science and clinical applications.

Vascular Birthmarks: Hemangiomas and Malformations. Mulliken JB, Young AE. Philadelphia, WB Saunders, 1988.

This comprehensive work contains beautifully illustrated examples of many orthopaedic syndromes such as Klippel-Trenaunay and Maffucci.

Genetic study of an orthopedic referral center. Hecht JT, Scott CI Jr. *J Pediatr Orthop* 1984;4:208-223.
>A prospective study at a pediatric referral hospital revealed that 25% of new patients and 46% of specialty clinic patients had orthopaedic diseases of genetic etiology.

An approach to the child with structural defects. Jones KL, Robinson LK. *J Pediatr Orthop* 1983;3:238-244.
>Presents a systematic approach to the child with congenital anomalies. This approach allows a specific overall diagnosis to be made.

Congenital malformations in 10,000 consecutive births in a university hospital: Need for genetic counseling and prenatal diagnosis. Van Regemorter N, Dodion J, Druart C, et al. *J Pediatr* 1984;104:386-390.
>An extensive analysis details the high birth incidence of generic and sporadic malformations, many of which are orthopaedic.

Hand-reduction malformations: Genetic and syndromic analysis. Pilarski RT, Pauli RM, Engber WD. *J Pediatr Orthop* 1985;5:274-280.
>Of 61 patients sequentially evaluated for congenital amputations of portions of the hand, 25% were the result of single gene disorders, and 33% had multiple malformation syndromes.

A comprehensive and critical assessment of overgrowth and overgrowth syndromes. Cohen MM Jr. *Adv Hum Genet* 1989;18:181-303,373-376.
>This comprehensive review article of overgrowth syndromes includes several of orthopaedic significance, such as Beckwith-Wiedemann syndrome, hemihypertrophy, and proteus syndrome.

Specific Conditions

Arthrogryposis Multiplex Congenita

Section I: Symposium. Arthrogryposis multiplex congenita. Thompson GH (ed). *Clin Orthop* 1985;194:2-123.
>This volume contains 15 articles covering all aspects of arthrogryposis. In addition to articles on management of hips, knees, feet, and upper extremities, it includes articles on the etiology of arthrogryposis (Swinyard CA, pp 15-29), genetic aspects (Hall JG, pp 44-53), neuropathology (Banker BQ, pp 30-43), and long-term outcome (Carlson WO, pp 115-123).

Talectomy in the treatment of resistant talipes equinovarus deformity in myelomeningocele and arthrogryposis. Dias LS, Stern LS. *J Pediatr Orthop* 1987;7:39-41.

Fourteen patients with spina bifida and four with arthrogryposis underwent talectomy after failed posterior-medial release. Effective hindfoot correction was achieved, but 25% required further surgery to correct forefoot adduction deformity.

Management of hip dislocations in children with arthrogryposis. Staheli LT, Chew DE, Elliott JS, et al. *J Pediatr Orthop* 1987;7:681-685.
> The medial approach was used to reduce dislocated hips in children with arthrogryposis. Stability was achieved, acetabular development was satisfactory, avascular necrosis was low (1 of 13 hips), and range of motion was better than in those treated by anterolateral incision or closed reduction.

Arthrogryposis of the hand. Yonenobu K, Tada K, Swanson AB. *J Pediatr Orthop* 1984;4:599-603.
> Analyzes patterns of hand deformity and the magnitude of resultant disability in 45 patients. Reviews the results of surgery in 17 cases. Surgery was very individualized.

Spinal deformities in patients with arthrogryposis: A review of 16 patients. Daher YH, Lonstein JE, Winter RB, et al. *Spine* 1985;10:609-613.
> Scoliosis in arthrogryposis was common, had variable patterns, was poorly controlled by an orthosis, and frequently required surgery, especially if thoracic lordosis was present.

Larsen Syndrome

Spinal deformities in Larsen's syndrome. Bowen JR, Ortega K, Ray S, et al. *Clin Orthop* 1985;197:159-163.
> A characteristic pattern of spinal deformity, including scoliosis and spondylolysis, was found in eight patients with Larsen syndrome. The cervical spine was the most severely involved area, with dysraphism and vertebral hypoplasia.

The Larsen syndrome occurring in four generations of one family. Stanley D, Seymour N. *Int Orthop* 1985;8:267-272.
> Eight patients with this syndrome are reviewed, with detailed emphasis on unique and complex foot deformities.

Early operation of the dislocated knee in Larsen's syndrome: A report of 2 cases. Munk S. *Acta Orthop Scand* 1988;59:582-584.
> Better than expected results in two patients with Larsen syndrome operated on before age 3 months lends support for early surgery of the dislocated knee.

Tracheomalacia and bronchomalacia associated with Larsen syndrome. Rock MJ, Green CG, Pauli RM, et al. *Pediatr Pulmonol* 1988;5:55-59.

Awareness of these airway abnormalities is helpful in avoiding anesthesia complications.

Freeman-Sheldon Whistling Face Syndrome

The whistling face syndrome, or craniocarpotarsal dysplasia: Report of two cases in a father and son and review of the literature. Malkawi H, Tarawneh M. *J Pediatr Orthop* 1983;3:364-369.
> Reviews this arthrogryposis-like syndrome involving hands and feet and notes that the characteristic deformities do not improve spontaneously, but require surgery.

Pterygium Syndromes

Limb pterygium syndromes: A review and report of eleven patients. Hall JG, Reed SD, Rosenbaum KN, et al. *Am J Med Genet* 1982;12:377-409.
> An introduction to the pterygium syndromes, multiple, popliteal, and lethal, with a word on genetics and associated findings.

Flexion contractures of the knee associated with popliteal webbing. Addison A, Webb PJ. *J Pediatr Orthop* 1983;3:376-379.
> The results and technique of surgical correction of the flexion deformity in 5 children with pterygium syndromes. Distinguishes between multiple pterygium syndrome and popliteal pterygium syndrome, and emphasizes the associated anatomic abnormalities.

Femoral shortening in correction of congenital knee flexion deformity with popliteal webbing. Saleh M, Gibson MF, Sharrard WJW. *J Pediatr Orthop* 1989;9:609-611.
> Outlines a technique to correct webbing by addressing both soft tissue and bone.

Congenital Contractural Arachnodactyly

Congenital contractural arachnodactyly: Report of a case and of an operation for knee contracture. Langenskiöld A. *J Bone Joint Surg* 1985;67B:44-46.
> Describes this syndrome, which can mimic Marfan syndrome, and gives a technique for managing the knee deformity.

Neurofibromatosis

Osseous manifestations of neurofibromatosis in childhood. Crawford AH Jr, Bagamery N. *J Pediatr Orthop* 1986;6:72-88.

A detailed review of the skeletal manifestations of neurofibromatosis in 116 children diagnosed before age 12 and followed for an average of five years.

Congenital pseudarthrosis of the forearm. Bayne LG. *Hand Clin* 1985;1:457-465.
>Four cases of pseudarthrosis of one or both bones of the forearm in patients with neurofibromatosis. Gives techniques for surgical management.

Congenital pseudarthrosis of the ulna: A report of two cases and a review of the literature. Ostrowski DM, Eilert RE, Waldstein G. *J Pediatr Orthop* 1985;5:463-467.
>Presents two cases of pseudarthrosis of the ulna in teenagers with neurofibromatosis and discusses treatment options.

Dystrophic spinal deformities in neurofibromatosis: Treatment by anterior and posterior fusion. Hsu LC, Lee PC, Leong JC. *J Bone Joint Surg* 1984;66B:495-499.
>Seven-year follow-up of 13 patients who underwent anterior/posterior combined fusion. Results were unsatisfactory in patients with sharply angled kyphoscoliosis, and good in those with smooth or minimal kyphosis.

Neurofibromatosis: A review of the clinical problem. Rubenstein AE. *Ann NY Acad Sci* 1986;486:1-13.
>A good review of the nonorthopaedic aspects of this disease.

The Proteus syndrome: The Elephant Man diagnosed. Tibbles JA, Cohen MM Jr. *Br Med J* 1986;293:683-685.
>Outlines the features of a condition previously misclassified as neurofibromatosis.

Proteus syndrome: An expanded phenotype. Clark RD, Donnai D, Rogers J, et al. *Am J Med Genet* 1987;27:99-117.
>Eleven patients with this syndrome illustrate the magnitude and the worsening of the physical findings, including the orthopaedic aspects of macrodactyly, gigantism, scoliosis, and exostosis.

Further diagnostic thoughts about the Elephant Man. Cohen MM Jr. *Am J Med Genet* 1988;29:777-782.
>Presents evidence that skeletal findings are more consistent with a diagnosis of proteus syndrome and hip trauma than with neurofibromatosis.

Down Syndrome

Atlantoaxial instability in individuals with Down syndrome: A fresh look at the evidence. Davidson RG. *Pediatrics* 1988;81:857-865.
> Reviews case histories of 31 persons with Down syndrome who went on to atlantoaxial dislocation. Concludes that routine roentgenographic screening unnecessarily restricts sports participation and does not prevent these neurologic catastrophes.

Atlantoaxial instability and Down syndrome. Pueschel SM. *Pediatrics* 1988;81:879-880.
> This editorial examines important, unresolved questions about Down syndrome, atlantoaxial instability, and Special Olympics.

Upper cervical ossicles in Down syndrome. French HG, Burke SW, Roberts JM, et al. *J Pediatr Orthop* 1987;7:69-71.
> Serial radiographs and radiographic anatomy in six young adults with Down syndrome suggest that the ossicles at C_2 represent an avulsion of the dens rather than a developmental ossiculum terminale.

Atlantoaxial instability in individuals with Down syndrome: Epidemiologic, radiographic, and clinical studies. Pueschel SM, Scola FH. *Pediatrics* 1987;80:555-560.
> Of 404 people with Down syndrome, 59 (14.6%) had C_1-C_2 instability. Of these, 53 were asymptomatic and six required fusion for myelopathy. An additional 95 patients followed longitudinally showed neither clinical nor roentgenographic changes.

Chronic atlanto-axial instability in Down syndrome. Burke SW, French HG, Roberts JM, et al. *J Bone Joint Surg* 1985;67A:1356-1360.
> Thirty-two Down patients had serial radiographs between 1970 and 1983. The average atlanto-dens interval increased, and, in seven, new instability developed.

Atlantoaxial instability in Down syndrome: Roentgenographic, neurologic, and somatosensory evoked potential studies. Pueschel SM, Findley TW, Furia J, et al. *J Pediatr* 1987;110:515-521.
> Compares asymptomatic Down syndrome patients with age-matched controls and a third group with symptomatic atlantoaxial instability. Mean spinal canal width differed in all 3 groups, and there was a high correspondence between somatosensory evoked potentials and atlanto-dens interval measurement.

Radiological screening for atlanto-axial instability in Down's syndrome. Jagjivan B, Spencer PA, Hosking G. *Clin Radiol* 1988;39:661-663.
> Of 220 Down patients of all ages, 15 (7%) had an abnormal atlanto-dens interval. Of these, 11 (70%) were under age 25.

Atlantoaxial instability and abnormalities of the odontoid in Down's syndrome. Elliott S, Morton RE, Whitelaw RA. *Arch Dis Child* 1988;63:1484-1489.

> In 67 children with Down syndrome, atlanto-dens instability was present in 7 (10%), odontoid hypoplasia in 15 (22%) and accessory odontoid ossicles in 2 (3%). In 94 adults with Down syndrome, instability was seen in 2 (2%), hypoplasia in 14 (15%), and ossicle in 2 (2%).

Down syndrome: Cervical spine abnormalities and problems. Van Dyke DC, Gahagan CA. *Clin Pediatr (Phila)* 1988;27:415-418.

> In 34 patients with Down syndrome, the most common cervical spine finding for those under age 21 was atlantoaxial instability. For those over age 25, it was significant degenerative arthritis.

Symptomatic atlantoaxial subluxation in persons with Down syndrome. Pueschel SM, Herndon JH, Gelch MM, et al. *J Pediatr Orthop* 1984;4:682-688.

> Reviews a prospective study of 40 patients with Down syndrome and atlantoaxial instability, including natural history and management of seven who exhibited neurologic compromise.

Lower cervical spondylosis and myelopathy in adults with Down's syndrome. Olive PM, Whitecloud TS III, Bennett JT. *Spine* 1988;13:781-784.

> In 105 Down patients with normal upper cervical spines, there was a significant prevalence of lower cervical degenerative changes and, in two patients, clinical myelopathy.

Atlantooccipital instability in Down syndrome. Rosenbaum DM, Blumhagen JD, King HA. *AJR* 1986;146:1269-1272.

> Two patients with striking atlanto-occipital instability on flexion/extension with a normal C1-C2 articulation.

Instability of the patellofemoral joint in Down syndrome. Dugdale TW, Renshaw TS. *J Bone Joint Surg* 1986;68A:405-413.

> Evaluates 210 institutionalized persons and 151 persons in the community with Down Syndrome. Less than 10% had dislocated/dislocatable patellae and only three were unable to walk because of patellofemoral instability.

Treatment of patellofemoral instability in Down's syndrome. Mendez AA, Keret D, MacEwen GD. *Clin Orthop* 1988;234:148-158.

> Sixteen Down patients with patellofemoral dislocations were reviewed. If initial ambulatory ability was either fair or good, nonsurgical management maintained or improved ambulatory status. But, if initial ambulatory ability was poor, then surgery was needed, and in those ambulation improved in 85%.

Management of dislocation of the hip in Down syndrome. Aprin H, Zink WP, Hall JE. *J Pediatr Orthop* 1985;5:428-431.

Reviews surgical treatment for dislocation of the hip in six patients with Down syndrome (ten hips). Those with dislocation and a normal acetabulum fared better than those with a dysplastic acetabulum.

Orthopedic disorders in school children with Down's syndrome with special reference to the incidence of joint laxity. Livingstone B, Hirst P. *Clin Orthop* 1986;207:74-76.
An analysis of orthopaedic problems and joint laxity in 39 school-age children with Down syndrome raised doubts as to whether ligament laxity is a major etiologic factor in joint problems in Down syndrome.

Down syndrome: Alzheimer's linked. Kolata G. *Science* 1985;230:1152-1153.
Notes the high frequency of precocious Alzheimer's disease in patients with Down syndrome and points out the implications.

de Lange Syndrome

Cornelia de Lange's syndrome: A review article (with emphasis on orthopedic significance). Joubin J, Pettrone CF, Pettrone FA. *Clin Orthop* 1982;171:180-185.
Six cases illustrate typical facial and skeletal features of this syndrome.

Progeria (Hutchinson-Gilford Syndrome)

Hip disease in Hutchinson-Gilford progeria syndrome. Gamble JG. *J Pediatr Orthop* 1984;4:585-589.
Progressive symptomatic hip subluxation/dislocation in two preadolescents with progeria.

Orthopaedic aspects of progeria. Moen C. *J Bone Joint Surg* 1982;64A:542-546.
Reviews two current cases and 60 in the literature. Emphasizes the progressive hip dysplasia, osteolysis, and avascular necrosis seen in this syndrome.

Familial Dysautonomia (Riley-Day Syndrome)

Physical therapy management of familial dysautonomia. Ganz SB, Levine DB, Axelrod FB, et al. *Phys Ther* 1983;63:1121-1124.
Outlines techniques to manage the spine deformity and postural contractures often seen in this syndrome.

Aseptic necrosis in familial dysautonomia. Mitnick JS, Axelrod FB, Genieser NB, et al. *Radiology* 1982;142:89-91.

Illustrates the avascular necrosis of femoral head, talus, and distal femur that occurs in as many as 8% of patients with this syndrome.

Scoliosis in familial dysautonomia. Robin GC. *Bull Hosp Jt Dis Orthop Inst* 1984;44:16-26.
An extensive review of surgical and nonsurgical management of the scoliosis and kyphosis that occur in 90% of patients with this syndrome.

Noonan Syndrome

Noonan syndrome. Allanson JE. *J Med Genet* 1987;24:9-13.
An extensive bibliography accompanies this overview of the Noonan syndrome. References to cases of malignant hyperthermia are of particular value.

Prader-Willi Syndrome

Prader-Willi syndrome. Cassidy SB. *Curr Probl Pediatr* 1984;14:1-55.
A monograph covering all aspects of this syndrome from historical notes to cytogenetics of chromosome 15, as well as management of the orthopaedic and nonorthopaedic manifestations.

Chromosome 15 in Prader-Willi syndrome. Fear CN, Mutton DE, Berry AC, et al. *Dev Med Child Neurol* 1985;27:305-311.
A structural deletion in the short arm of chromosome 15 is present in half the patients diagnosed with Prader-Willi syndrome.

Fetal Alcohol Syndrome

Alcohol teratogenicity in the human: A detailed assessment of specificity, critical period, and threshold. Ernhart CB, Sokol RJ, Martier S, et al. *Am J Obstet Gynecol* 1987;156:33-39.
A detailed prospective study of 359 neonates revealed that the critical period for alcohol teratogenicity is around the time of conception, and that certain anomalies, but not all, occur in a dose-response manner.

Bone fusion in the foetal alcohol syndrome. Jaffer Z, Nelson M, Beighton P. *J Bone Joint Surg* 1981;63B:569-571.
Carpal fusions and radio-ulnar synostosis were found in three of 15 patients with fetal alcohol syndrome.

The orthopedic aspects of the fetal alcohol syndrome. Spiegel PG, Pekman WM, Rich BH, et al. *Clin Orthop* 1979;139:58-63.
Cervical spine fusions, radio-ulnar synostosis, and contractures are the common orthopaedic complications of this syndrome.

Independent dysmorphology evaluations at birth and 4 years of age for children exposed to varying amounts of alcohol in utero. Graham JM Jr, Hanson JW, Darby BL, et al. *Pediatrics* 1988;81:772-778.

> The greater the levels of alcohol exposure during early pregnancy, the more likely the child will have recognizable, persistent fetal alcohol effects.

Fetal AIDS Syndrome

Fetal AIDS syndrome score: Correlation between severity of dysmorphism and age at diagnosis of immunodeficiency. Marion RW, Wiznia AA, Hutcheon RG, et al. *Am J Dis Child* 1987;141:429-431.

> Characteristic dysmorphic facial features of children born with HIV infection are evaluated in 37 children and found to have been helpful in establishing the diagnosis prior to clinical AIDS.

Rett Syndrome

Rett syndrome: Natural history in 70 cases. Naidu S, Murphy M, Moser HW, et al. *Am J Med Genet* 1986;24(suppl 1):61-72.

> A review of all aspects of this syndrome in 70 females ages 2-1/2 to 34 years, with emphasis on the time of appearance and severity of each characteristic. This is one of 40 articles in this supplement volume devoted to Rett syndrome.

Orthopedic aspects of Rett syndrome: A multicenter review. Loder RT, Lee CL, Richards BS. *J Pediatr Orthop* 1989;9:557-562.

> In a review of 36 patients with Rett Syndrome, two thirds had orthopaedic problems, of which spinal deformity (45%) and joint contractures (36%) were the most frequent.

TAR (Thrombocytopenia With Absent Radii) Syndrome

Dysplasia of the knee associated with the syndrome of thrombocytopenia and absent radius. Schoenecker PL, Cohn AK, Sedgwick WG, et al. *J Bone Joint Surg* 1984;66A:421-427.

> Eighteen of 21 patients with thrombocytopenia with absent radii had developmental anomalies of the lower extremity and significant deformity of the knee. Details the difficulties of treatment.

VATER (Vertebral, Anal, Tracheoesophageal, Renal, and Radial Limb Anomalies) Association

Orthopaedic aspects of the VATER association. Lawhon SM, MacEwen GD, Bunnell WP. *J Bone Joint Surg* 1986;68A:424-429.

A review of 28 patients with the VATER association (vertebral, anal, tracheoesophageal, renal, and radial limb anomalies), with details of 12 who required either spine or upper extremity surgery.

Femoral Hypoplasia-Unusual Facies

The femoral hypoplasia-unusual facies syndrome. Burn J, Winter RM, Baraitser M, et al. *J Med Genet* 1984;21:331-340.
> Features of this syndrome are delineated, including the dysgenesis of the proximal femur, the elbow, and the lumbar spine.

Femoral hypoplasia-unusual facies syndrome in infants of diabetic mothers. Johnson JP, Carey JC, Gooch WM III, et al. *J Pediatr* 1983;102:866-872.
> The etiologic relationship of this syndrome to maternal diabetes is discussed.

Congenital deficiency of the femur. Kalamchi A, Cowell HR, Kim KI. *J Pediatr Orthop* 1985;5:129-134.
> Reviews patients with femoral deficiency, some of whom had this syndrome, although they are not specifically so identified.

Connective Tissue Disorders

Biochemistry and Classifications

Molecular basis of clinical heterogeneity in the Ehlers-Danlos syndrome. Byers PH, Holbrook KA. *Ann NY Acad Sci* 1985;460:298-310.
> A valuable review of the biochemical and genetic aspects of ten of the Ehlers-Danlos syndromes.

Biochemistry of collagen in diseases. Uitto J, Murray LW, Blumberg B, et al. *Ann Intern Med* 1986;105:740-756.
> Reviews the biochemistry of collagen, highlighting specific molecular alterations and their corresponding clinical disease.

The differential symptomatology of errors of collagen metabolism: A tentative classification. Maroteaux P, Frézal J, Cohen-Solal L. *Am J Med Genet* 1986;24:219-230.
> This classification schema addresses the specific collagen in skin, joints, bone, and blood vessels and corresponding disease entities.

Genetic disorders of collagen. Tsipouras P, Ramirez F. *J Med Genet* 1987;24:2-8.
> Reviews biochemical and molecular differences that account for the clinical features of Ehlers-Danlos, Marfan, and osteogenesis imperfecta.

Inherited collagen disorders. Sykes B. *Mol Biol Med* 1989;6:19-26.

> A sophisticated article dealing with the structure of collagen, the genes that control its manufacture, and the mutant genes responsible for its abnormalities. Discusses prenatal diagnosis of collagen diseases.

Marfan

Dural ectasia is a common feature of the Marfan syndrome. Pyeritz RE, Fishman EK, Bernhardt BA, et al. *Am J Hum Genet* 1988;43:726-732.
> Widening of the lumbar spinal canal is present in two thirds of patients with Marfan syndrome, some of whom had associated pedicle erosion, meningocele, and neurologic signs.

Iatrogenic kyphosis: A complication of Harrington instrumentation in Marfan's syndrome. A case report. Amis J, Herring JA. *J Bone Joint Surg* 1984;66A:460-464.
> Reports complications of managing scoliosis in patients with ligamentous laxity syndromes.

Homocystinuria

The natural history of homocystinuria due to cystathionine beta-synthase deficiency. Mudd SH, Skovby F, Levy HL, et al. *Am J Hum Genet* 1985;37:1-31.
> A study of 629 patients with homocystinuria detailing the onset and natural history of the most common complications (osteoporosis, thromboembolism, optic lens dislocation). Comparison is made between B-6 (pyridoxine) responsive and nonresponsive individuals.

Homocystinuria versus Marfan's syndrome: The therapeutic relevance of the differential diagnosis. Boers GH, Polder TW, Cruysberg JR, et al. *Neth J Med* 1984;27:206-212.
> This article contains a lucid discussion of the biochemistry and the rationale for treatment, and has excellent patient photographs. It is worth having the library search for it.

Homocystinuria: Clinical, biochemical and genetic aspects of cystathionine beta-synthase and its deficiency in man. Skovby F. *Acta Paediatr Scand* 1985;321(suppl):1-21.
> An excellent review of the entire subject, including clinical features, but mainly details about the biochemistry and the rationale for therapy.

Osteogenesis Imperfecta

Osteogenesis imperfecta. Gertner JM, Root L. *Orthop Clin North Am* 1990;21:151-162.

A review of this group of fragile bone syndromes including an up-to-date classification, collagen biochemistry, treatment, and prenatal diagnosis.

Third international conference on osteogenesis imperfecta. Cetta G, Ramirez F, Tsipouras P (eds). *Ann NY Acad Sci* 1988;543:1-185.
> This volume, devoted to osteogenesis imperfecta, has 21 articles by leaders in the field. They cover such wide ranging topics as: Nosology and genetics (Sillence DO, pp 1-15); clinical heterogenicity (Maroteaux P, pp 16-29); collagen biochemistry (Hollister DW, pp 62-72); the molecular basis of clinical disease (Byers PH, pp 117-128); prenatal diagnosis (Sykes B, pp 136-141); and orthopaedic and medical treatment (Cole WG, pp 157-166; Finidori G, pp 167-169; and Brunelli PC, pp 170-179).

Consequences of an osteogenesis imperfecta diagnosis for survival and ambulation. Shapiro F. *J Pediatr Orthop* 1985;5:456-462.
> A comparison of survival and ambulation of patients with osteogenesis imperfecta when the time of initial fracture (birth, prewalking, postambulation) is considered.

- Psychosocial aspects of osteogenesis imperfecta. Shea-Landry GL, Cole DE. *Can Med Assoc J* 1986;135:977-981.
> This article considers the emotional, social, and financial burdens placed upon osteogenesis imperfecta patients and their families.

Non-union of fractures in children who have osteogenesis imperfecta. Gamble JG, Rinsky LA, Strudwick J, et al. *J Bone Joint Surg* 1988;70A:439-443.
> Of 52 patients with osteogenesis imperfecta, 10 had 12 nonunions, all of which resulted in functional disability.

Osteogenesis imperfecta: Comprehensive management. Marini JC. *Adv Pediatr* 1988;35:391-426.
> In addition to a lucid discussion of classification, collagen biochemistry, and orthopaedic management, there are also details of caring for the associated neurologic, ocular, hearing, dental, growth, and cardiovascular problems.

Osteogenesis imperfecta: Perspectives. Stoltz MR, Dietrich SL, Marshall GJ. *Clin Orthop* 1989;242:120-136.
> A comprehensive review of this heterogenous group of disorders with an emphasis on pediatric and orthopaedic management.

Fracture failure mechanisms in patients with osteogenesis imperfecta. Alman B, Frasca P. *J Orthop Res* 1987;5:139-143.
> Biomechanical data revealed osteogenesis imperfecta bone to be more plastic ("taffy") with decreased work to failure.

Complications of intramedullary rods in osteogenesis imperfecta: Bailey-Dubow rods versus nonelongating rods. Gamble JG, Strudwick WJ, Rinsky LA, et al. *J Pediatr Orthop* 1988;8:645-649.

> A review of 108 intramedullary roddings in 29 patients with osteogenesis imperfecta revealed that although non-elongating rods had a higher reoperation and replacement rate than Bailey-Dubow rods, Bailey-Dubow rods had a higher overall complication rate.

Ehlers Danlos (Type IV)

Clinical presentations of Ehlers Danlos syndrome type IV. Pope FM, Narcisi P, Nicholls AC, et al. *Arch Dis Child* 1988;63:1016-1025.

> A comprehensive review of this vascular type of Ehlers-Danlos syndrome, including prenatal diagnosis, early clinical identification, and natural history.

Skeletal Dysplasias

Atlas of Skeletal Dysplasias. Wynne-Davies R, Hall CM, Apley AG. Edinburgh, Churchill Livingstone, 1985.

> Superbly organized, with a logical classification, just enough text, and outstanding examples of each bone dysplasia from infancy to adulthood.

Inherited Disorders of the Skeleton, ed 2. Beighton P. Edinburgh, Churchill Livingstone, 1988.

> Somewhat narrower in scope than the previous text, but offers a thorough discussion of many of the dysplasias and other conditions of the skeleton seen in infancy and childhood.

The prevalence of skeletal dysplasias: An estimate of their minimum frequency and the number of patients requiring orthopaedic care. Wynne-Davies R, Gormley J. *J Bone Joint Surg* 1985;67B:133-137.

> Estimates that during the period 1950-1979 there were 10,000 individuals in Britain with skeletal dysplasias, of whom 6,000 required substantial orthopaedic care.

The birth prevalence rates for the skeletal dysplasias. Orioli IM, Castilla EE, Barbosa-Neto JG. *J Med Genet* 1986;23:328-332.

> From 1978 through 1983 there were 2.3 skeletal dysplasias per 10,000 births in Latin America, with achondroplasia the most common. An argument is made that this is an underestimation by 50%.

Congenital generalised bone dysplasias: A clinical, radiological, and epidemiological survey. Andersen PE Jr, Hauge M. *J Med Genet* 1989;26:37-44.

> The prevalence of skeletal dysplasias from 1970 through 1983 in Denmark was found to be greater than previously assumed, with

achondroplasia less common than multiple epiphyseal dysplasia and others.

Orthopaedic aspects of skeletal dysplasias. Bassett GS. In Greene WB (ed): American Academy of Orthopaedic Surgeons *Instructional Course Lectures, XXXIX*. Park Ridge, IL, American Academy of Orthopaedic Surgeons, 1990, pp 381-387.
Lower-extremity abnormalities in dwarfing conditions. Bassett GS. In Greene WB (ed): American Academy of Orthopaedic Surgeons *Instructional Course Lectures, XXXIX*. Park Ridge, IL, American Academy of Orthopaedic Surgeons, 1990, pp 389-397.
Spinal deformity in short-stature syndromes. Tolo VT. In Greene WB (ed): American Academy of Orthopaedic Surgeons *Instructional Course Lectures, XXXIX*. Park Ridge, IL, American Academy of Orthopaedic Surgeons, 1990, pp 399-405.
> These three articles outline the abnormalities and treatment options in the skeletal dysplasias most frequently treated by an orthopaedic surgeon.

Achondroplasia

Lengthening of the lower limbs in achondroplastic patients: A comparative study of four techniques. Aldegheri R, Trivella G, Renzi-Brivio L, et al. *J Bone Joint Surg* 1988;70B:69-73.
> The results of limb lengthening in 61 patients with achondroplasia and 11 with hypochondroplasia is presented with details of length achieved, healing time, and complications.

Cervicomedullary compression in young patients with achondroplasia: Value of comprehensive neurologic and respiratory evaluation. Reid CS, Pyeritz RE, Kopits SE, et al. *J Pediatr* 1987;110:522-530.
> A study of 26 young patients with achondroplasia showing that 85% had respiratory abnormalities, nine of which were caused by cervicomedullary cord compression.

Human Achondroplasia: A Multidisciplinary Approach. Nicoletti B, Kopits SE, Ascani E, et al (eds). New York, Plenum Press, 1988.
> The papers in this volume, submitted by the participants at the First International Conference on Human Achondroplasia in Rome in 1986, elaborate in more detail the proceedings from that conference. The 59 papers deal with basic genetics and histochemistry, orthopaedic aspects, spinal disorders, limb lengthening, anesthesia problems, and social and psychological considerations.

Pseudoachondroplasia

Pseudoachondroplasia: Clinical diagnosis at different ages and comparison of autosomal dominant and recessive types. A review of 32 patients (26 kindreds). Wynne-Davies R, Hall CM, Young ID. *J Med Genet* 1986;23:425-434.
> Using mainly radiographic material, the natural history of pseudoachondroplasia from infancy to adulthood is illustrated.

Multiple Epiphyseal Dysplasia

Bilateral femoral head dysplasia and osteochondritis: Multiple epiphyseal dysplasia tarda, spondylo-epiphyseal dysplasia tarda, and bilateral Legg-Perthes disease. Andersen PE Jr, Schantz K, Bollerslev J, et al. *Acta Radiol* 1988;29:705-709.
> In addition to determining a population prevalence of these conditions, the distinguishing radiographic characteristics are illustrated, thus reducing the likelihood of misdiagnosis.

Spondyloepiphyseal Dysplasia

Spondylo-epiphyseal dysplasia tarda: The X-linked variety in three brothers. Iceton JA, Horne G. *J Bone Joint Surg* 1986;68B:616-619.
> The clinical features of this type of spondyloepiphyseal dysplasia are reviewed, stressing the variable severity of hip osteoarthritis from chronic and mild to acute and disabling.

Spondyloepiphyseal dysplasia tarda: Report of a family with autosomal dominant transmission. Schantz K, Andersen PE Jr, Justesen P. *Acta Orthop Scand* 1988;59:716-719.
> A well illustrated report of three members of a family with the autosomal dominant form of spondyloepiphyseal dysplasia tarda.

Enchondromatosis

The malignant potential of enchondromatosis. Schwartz HS, Zimmerman NB, Simon MA, et al. *J Bone Joint Surg* 1987;69A:269-274.
> Analyzes the types of malignant skeletal and nonskeletal tumors in 37 patients with Ollier disease and 7 with Maffucci syndrome, and calculates life survival rates.

Chondrosarcoma in Maffucci's syndrome. Sun TC, Swee RG, Shives TC, et al. *J Bone Joint Surg* 1985;67A:1214-1219.
> Based on nine patients, five of whom had chondrosarcoma, and a review of the literature, an incidence of malignant degeneration is calculated at 18%.

Multiple Hereditary Exostosis

Management of deformities of the forearm in multiple hereditary osteochondromas. Fogel GR, McElfresh EC, Peterson HA, et al. *J Bone Joint Surg* 1984;66A:670-680.
>This article describes the results of surgical treatment in 18 patients. Early excision of the osteochondroma by itself did not alter progression of the deformity. Distal radial hemiepiphyseal stapling with ulnar lengthening was usually necessary if radio-carpal angulation or subluxation of the lunate had occurred. Deformities of the forearm in these patients required early and aggressive therapy to prevent disability.

Visualization by dynamic and static osseous scintigraphy of pelvic chondrosarcoma in multiple hereditary exostosis. Jackson RL, Llaurado JG. *Clin Nucl Med* 1987;12:113-115.
>Compares the Tc99m MDP flow and blood pool scintigrams with the "bone scan" in a patient with a low grade chondrosarcoma.

The infrequency of malignant disease in diaphyseal aclasis and neurofibromatosis. Voutsinas S, Wynne-Davies R. *J Med Genet* 1983;20:345-349.
>A review of both index patients and their relatives places a more reasonable figure for malignant change in multiple hereditary exostosis at 0.5% and in neurofibromatosis at 2.0%. Both figures are lower than previous estimates.

The treatment of hereditary multiple exostosis of the upper extremity. Wood VE, Sauser D, Mudge D. *J Hand Surg* 1985;10A:505-513.
>Of 50 patients with this dysplasia, 30 had significant arm deformities. Details results and options of treatment in 10 patients.

Camptomelic Dysplasia

Spinal abnormalities in camptomelic dysplasia. Coscia MF, Bassett GS, Bowen JR, et al. *J Pediatr Orthop* 1989;9:6-14.
>Severe scoliosis (average 63 degrees) and severe hyperkyphosis (average 126 degrees) are present in the majority of patients with this bone dysplasia. Requires aggressive treatment because survival is longer than previously expected.

Mucopolysaccharidosis (Morquio)

Clinical findings in 12 patients with MPS IVA (Morquio's disease): Further evidence for heterogeneity. Part I: Clinical and biochemical findings. Nelson J, Broadhead D, Mossman J. *Clin Genet* 1988;33:111-120.
>Twelve patients with MPS IV-A all had N-acetyl galactosamine-6-sulphate sulphatase deficiency. Variations in residual enzyme activity

25

were postulated as the reason for differences in severity of physical findings.

Clinical findings in 12 patients with MPS IVA (Morquio's disease): Further evidence for heterogeneity. Part III: Odontoid dysplasia. Nelson J, Thomas PS. *Clin Genet* 1988;33:126-130.
> Odontoid dysplasia was present in all. The magnitude of atlanto-axial instability varied, however, and correlated with overall clinical severity.

Nail Patella Syndrome

Foot deformities associated with onycho-osteodysplasia: A familial study and a review of associated features. Høgh J, Macnicol MF. *Int Orthop* 1985;9:135-138.
> Cases are presented where rigid clubfoot and calcaneovalgus feet are part of this syndrome.

Long-term follow-up of the treatment of a family with nail-patella syndrome. Yakish SD, Fu FH. *J Pediatr Orthop* 1983;3:360-363.
> Ten-year follow-up of four patients who underwent quadricepsplasty for subluxing patella, and five-year follow-up of two patients who underwent radial head resection for dislocation.

Pycnodysostosis

Pycnodysostosis. Mills KL, Johnston AW. *J Med Genet* 1988;25:550-553.
> This case report includes good radiographs, a discussion of diagnosis, and a pertinent bibliography.

Infantile Cortical Hyperostosis

Pathology of infantile cortical hyperostosis (Caffey's disease): Report of a case. Pazzaglia UE, Byers PD, Beluffi G, et al. *J Bone Joint Surg* 1985;67A:1417-1426.
> Provides detailed pathologic specimens and discusses a florid case of Caffey's disease that ended in death. An inflammatory process is implicated.

Infantile cortical hyperostosis with osteomyelitis of the humerus. Blasier RB, Aronson DD. *J Pediatr Orthop* 1985;5:222-224.
> The coincidence of Caffey's disease and osteomyelitis led to a delay in diagnosis of the bone infection.

Infantile cortical hyperostosis with intramedullary lesions. Leung VC, Lee KE. *J Pediatr Orthop* 1985;5:354-357.

It is suggested that intramedullary lytic lesions are also a part of the roentgenographic appearance of Caffey's disease.

Caffey's disease: Nuclear medicine and radiologic correlation. A case of mistaken identity. Tien R, Barron BJ, Dhekne RD. *Clin Nucl Med* 1988;13:583-585.
>Caffey's disease was mistaken for child abuse. The role of bone scanning is discussed.

Fibrous Dysplasia

Fibrous dysplasia of the spine. Wright JF, Stoker DJ. *Clin Radiol* 1988;39:523-527.
>Presents radiologic features of 11 cases of fibrous dysplasia of the spine.

Monostotic fibrous dysplasia of the lumbar spine: Case report and review of the literature. Troop JK, Herring JA. *J Pediatr Orthop* 1988;8:599-601.
>Involvement of the spine with monostotic fibrous dysplasia rather than the more common polyostotic.

Multiple osteotomies with Zickel nail fixation for polyostotic fibrous dysplasia involving the proximal part of the femur. Freeman BH, Bray EW III, Meyer LC. *J Bone Joint Surg* 1987;69A:691-698.
>The natural history of fibrous dysplasia of the proximal femur is reviewed in four patients (six femurs). Treatment by osteotomies and Zickel nail resulted in relief of pain, no further fractures, and no recurrence of deformity in 75%.

Fibrous dysplasia of the femoral neck: Treatment by cortical bone-grafting. Enneking WF, Gearen PF. *J Bone Joint Surg* 1986;68A:1415-1422.
>Successful treatment of 15 patients (aged 11 to 32) with symptomatic fibrous dysplasia of the femoral neck by using autologous fibula cortical grafts without curettage or internal fixation.

Desmoplastic fibroma arising in fibrous dysplasia: Chromosomal analysis and review of the literature. Bridge JA, Rosenthal H, Sanger WG, et al. *Clin Orthop* 1989;247:272-278.
>Reviews the association of this rare tumor with fibrous dysplasia and the findings of chromosomal aberrations in benign tumors.

Cystic degeneration of fibrous dysplasia masquerading as sarcoma. Simpson AH, Creasy TS, Williamson DM, et al. *J Bone Joint Surg* 1989;71B:434-436.
>Three patients (adults) had rapidly enlarging areas of known fibrous dysplasia that turned out to be cystic degeneration although they presented as malignancy. Magnetic resonance imaging was helpful.

Adamantinoma of the tibia masked by fibrous dysplasia: Report of three cases. Schajowicz F, Santini-Araujo E. *Clin Orthop* 1989;238:294-301.

> Three cases of adamantinoma appeared in tibiae with the typical features of fibrous dysplasia (in 1 case) and osteofibrous dysplasia of Campanacci (in 2 cases).

Osteosarcoma in fibrous dysplasia. Taconis WK. *Skeletal Radiol* 1988;17:163-170.

> Two cases of osteosarcomatous transformation plus a calculation from the Netherlands Tumor Committee that the incidence of sarcomatous transformation is 0.5% (which still may be too high).

Malignant transformation of fibrous dysplasia: A case report and review of the literature. Yabut SM Jr, Kenan S, Sissons HA, et al. *Clin Orthop* 1988;228:281-289.

> One new case, plus a review of the 83 cases in the literature, of malignant transformation in fibrous dysplasia. Osteosarcoma was the most common type; craniofacial bones the most common site.

MRI findings in osteofibrous dysplasia. Dominguez R, Saucedo J, Fenstermacher M. *Magn Reson Imaging* 1989;7:567-570.

> Magnetic resonance imaging signal characteristics are able to distinguish fibrous dysplasia from osteofibrous dysplasia of Campanacci.

MR appearance of fibrous dysplasia. Utz JA, Kransdorf MJ, Jelinek JS, et al. *J Comput Assist Tomogr* 1989;13:845-851.

> The appearance of magnetic resonance imaging of fibrous dysplasia in 11 anatomic sites is reviewed. The T-1 weighted image has a decreased signal intensity, but the T-2 weighted signal is variable.

Scintigraphic manifestation of fibrous dysplasia. Machida K, Makita K, Nishikawa J, et al. *Clin Nucl Med* 1986;11:426-429.

> Fifty-nine lesions in 26 patients were studied using Tc99m medronate methylene diphosphonate scintigraphy. In spite of obvious changes on plain roentgenograms, 14% of cystic lesions and 7% of ground glass lesions had no uptake.

Fibrous dysplasia: An analysis of options for treatment. Stephenson RB, London MD, Hankin FM, et al. *J Bone Joint Surg* 1987;69A:400-409.

> Reviews the results of treatment of 65 lesions in 43 patients. Closed treatment of symptomatic lesions of the upper extremity was satisfactory in 93%. In the lower extremity, results were highly age-dependent, with those under the age of 18 rarely having a satisfactory result from either closed or open treatment.

McCune-Albright syndrome: Long-term follow-up. Lee PA, Van Dop C, Migeon CJ. *JAMA* 1986;256:2980-2984.

Fifteen patients with McCune-Albright Syndrome were followed clinically into adulthood. Fractures only occurred during childhood, but hearing impairment and some endocrinopathy were present in adults.

Ultrastructure of fibrous dysplasia of bone: A study of its fibrous, osseous, and cartilaginous components. Greco MA, Steiner GC. *Ultrastruct Pathol* 1986;10:55-66.

A detailed analysis of the electron and light microscopy findings in 8 cases of fibrous dysplasia.

Estrogen receptors in bone in a patient with polyostotic fibrous dysplasia (McCune-Albright syndrome). Kaplan FS, Fallon MD, Boden SD, et al. *N Engl J Med* 1988;319:421-425.

Estrogen and progesterone tissue receptors were found in osteogenic cells from fibrous dysplasia lesions. Questions are raised regarding hormonal effects and other factors controlling growth of the skeleton.

Metabolic Bone Disease

Rickets, osteomalacia, and renal osteodystrophy: An update. Mankin HJ. *Orthop Clin North Am* 1990;21:81-96.

A summary of the subject with emphasis on recent knowledge, including the causes of rachitic syndromes, the homeostatic mechanisms for calcium and phosphorus as well as clinical, roentgenographic, and therapeutic considerations of rickets and renal osteodystrophy.

Calcium homeostasis. Boden SD, Kaplan FS. *Orthop Clin North Am* 1990;21:31-42.

Reviews calcium physiology, both intra- and extracellular, and the calcium-regulating hormones.

The physiology of the vitamin D endocrine system. Audran M, Gross M, Kumar R. *Semin Nephrol* 1986;6:4-20.

The role of vitamin D in maintaining calcium and phosphate homeostasis and the effects of vitamin D on cellular differentiation.

The vitamin D story: A collaborative effort of basic science and clinical medicine. DeLuca HF. *FASEB J* 1988;2:224-236.

Vitamin D, from its discovery in 1919 to the biochemical synthesis of 1,25 dehydroxy D and its clinical applications along the way.

Rickets

The X-linked hypophosphatemic vitamin D resistant rickets: Old and new concepts. Brunette MG. *Int J Pediatr Nephrol* 1985;6:55-62.

Gives the biochemistry and clinical management of the most common of the vitamin D-resistant rickets. (This journal may be hard to find.)

Hypophosphatemic rickets: Still misdiagnosed and inadequately treated. Greene WB, Kahler SG. *South Med J* 1985;78:1179-1184.
Surgical aspects of limb deformity in hypophosphatemic rickets. Greene WB, Kahler SG. *South Med J* 1985;78:1185-1189.

> These two articles analyze the presentation and results of medical therapy in 25 children and the results of surgical therapy in 17 operations. The diagnosis was typically delayed with resultant skeletal deformity. Medical therapy did not change limb alignment. Results of surgery were improved by adequate medical therapy, osteotomies at or near completion of growth, and use of the mechanical axis to plan the reconstructive procedure.

Clinical features of hereditary resistance to 1,25-dihydroxyvitamin D (hereditary hypocalcemic vitamin D resistant rickets type II). Liberman UA, Eil C, Marx SJ. *Adv Exp Med Biol* 1986;196:391-406.

> An inborn error of vitamin D metabolism in which rickets is the result of end organ resistance to 1,25 dihydroxyvitamin D.

Effects of anticonvulsant drug therapy on bone mineral density in a pediatric population. Timperlake RW, Cook SD, Thomas KA, et al. *J Pediatr Orthop* 1988;8:467-470.

> In spite of the recognized association of rickets in children with epilepsy, the authors were unable to document differences in bone mineral density in 20 epileptic children and matched controls.

Hereditary tubular disorders of the Fanconi type and the idiopathic Fanconi syndrome. Bickel H, Manz F. *Prog Clin Biol Res* 1989;305:111-135.

> Itemizes the various hereditary and acquired diseases with dysfunction of the proximal renal tubule, glucosuria, aminoaciduria, and rickets.

Rickets of prematurity: Controversies in causation and prevention. Campbell DE, Fleischman AR. *Clin Perinatol* 1988;15:879-890.

> Metabolic bone disease, a common disorder of premature infants, is thought to be caused by inadequate intake of calcium or phosphorus over an extended period of time.

Renal Osteodystrophy

The wide spectrum of renal osteodystrophy in children. Wolfson BJ, Capitanio MA. *CRC Crit Rev Diagn Imaging* 1987;27:297-319.

> Reviews the bone changes of renal osteodystrophy in children and the changes that come from treatment. Well illustrated.

Hypophosphatasia

Analysis of liver/bone/kidney alkaline phosphatase mRNA, DNA, and enzymatic activity in cultured skin fibroblasts from 14 unrelated patients with

severe hypophosphatasia. Weiss MJ, Ray K, Fallon MD, et al. *Am J Hum Genet* 1989;44:686-694.
>   An attempt to understand the gene defects that result in the defective bone mineralization in this heritable disorder.

Chronic idiopathic hyperphosphatasia and fibrous dysplasia in the same child. Pazzaglia UE, Barbieri D, Beluffi G, et al. *J Pediatr Orthop* 1989;9:709-716.
>   A well documented case (clinical, radiographic, and histologic) of hyperphosphatasia is presented. The coincident occurrence of mandibular fibrous dysplasia raises questions of an underlying common defect in control of bone-cell activity.

Hyperostosis With Hyperphosphatemia

Hyperostosis with hyperphosphatemia: A case report and review of the literature. Talab YA, Mallouh A. *J Pediatr Orthop* 1988;8:338-341.
>   A review of the unusual combination of attacks of bone pain and limb swelling, periosteal reaction, and increased serum phosphorus with normal calcium and parathormone.

Juvenile Osteoporosis

Effect of calcitonin replacement therapy in idiopathic juvenile osteoporosis. Jackson EC, Strife CF, Tsang RC, et al. *Am J Dis Child* 1988;142:1237-1239.
>   Injections of calcitonin both with and without the addition of oral calcitriol and oral calcium failed to reduce the number of fractures, nor did it alter the excessive bone resorption seen at biopsy.

Characteristics and bisphosphonate treatment of a patient with juvenile osteoporosis. Hoekman K, Papapoulos SE, Peters AC, et al. *J Clin Endocrinol Metab* 1985;61:952-956.
>   There was striking improvement in clinical symptoms, calcium balance, and roentgenograms following treatment with a bisphosphonate capable of inhibiting bone resorption.

Pediatric Cervical Spine

Peter D. Pizzutillo, MD
Eric Jones, MD

The cervical spine. Hensinger RN, Fielding JW. In Morrissy RT (ed): *Pediatric Orthopaedics*, ed 3. Philadelphia, JB Lippincott, 1990.

Congenital malformations. In Shreck H (ed): The Cervical Spine Research Society, Editorial Committee: *The Cervical Spine*, ed 2. Philadelphia, JB Lippincott, 1989, pp 226-285.

The Upper Cervical Spine. von Torklus D, Gehle W. New York, Grune & Stratton, 1972.
> Detailed reference source for upper cervical anomalies.

Basilar Impression

Basilar impression and Arnold-Chiari malformation: A study of 66 cases. De Barros MC, Farias W, Ataíde L, et al. *J Neurol Neurosurg Psychiat* 1968;31:596-605.
> This unique clinical experience allows comparisons of the two conditions.

The significance of abnormalities of the cervical spine. McRae DL. *Am J Roentgen* 1960;84:3-25.
> This lecture, given to the American Roentgen Ray Society, covers everything from congenital anomalies to cervical disk disease and osteoarthritis. Although most of the patients presented are adults, many of the abnormalities are ones that can be discovered in childhood. The article is very specific in reviewing neurologic symptoms and signs in patients with radiographic abnormalities of the cervical spine. The conclusion is to correlate clinical and radiographic findings to help determine which patients require treatment.

Basilar impression (platybasia): A bizarre developmental anomaly of the occipital bone and upper cervical spine with striking and misleading neurologic manifestations. Chamberlain WE. *Yale J Biol Med* 1939;11:487-496.
> Classic.

Occipitoatlantal Complex

Occipito-atlantal instability in children: A report of five cases and review of the literature. Georgopoulos G, Pizzutillo PD, Lee MS. *J Bone Joint Surg* 1987;69A:429-436.
> Occipitoatlantal instability is most commonly associated with trauma. Presents nontraumatic group of patients with instability and bizarre vertebrobasilar signs. Surgical stabilization is recommended for both traumatic and nontraumatic forms of occipitoatlantal instability.

Anomalies of the occipitocervical articulation. Nicholson JT, Sherk HH. *J Bone Joint Surg* 1968;50A:295-304.
> This article reviews the embryology and radiology of the occipital cervical articulation. The three types of anomalies described include congenital atlanto-occipital fusion, accessory vertebral elements between the atlas and the occiput, and anomalies of the apex of the odontoid process. Signs and symptoms of these anomalies become evident most often in young adults who present with weakness, ataxia, suboccipital and neck pain, and progressive tetraparesis. Surgical treatment is often needed.

Occipitalization of the atlas. McRae DL, Barnum AS. *Am J Roentgen* 1953;70:23-46.
> Covers 25 cases of various forms of occipitalization. Although only one of the patients is a child, the adult patients had their occipitalization on a congenital basis. Presentation typically included a significant amount of neurologic involvement, notably weakness and ataxia of the lower extremities, numbness, and pain. Occipital headaches and blurring vision may also occur. Radiographically, the cervical-occipital region should be evaluated by flexion and extension views as well as other special studies to determine instability and spinal cord compression.

Bony abnormalities in the region of the foramen magnum: Correlation of the anatomic and neurologic findings. McRae DL. *Acta Radiol* 1953;40:335-355.
> Reviews over 100 adults with bony abnormalities in the region of the foramen magnum. These patients were identified in a study of patients with syringomyelia and syringobulbia, 40% of whom had bony abnormalities in the region of the foramen magnum, most commonly occipitalization of the atlas and platybasia with basilar invagination. Other anomalies noted were an odontoid process separate from the axis and chronic atlantoaxial dislocation.

Atlantoaxial Instability

Normal sagittal diameter and variation in the pediatric cervical spine.
Yousefzadeh DK, El-Khoury GY, Smith WL. *Radiology* 1982;144:319-325.
> A gradual widening of the sagittal diameter of the lower cervical canal and even ballooning in the mid-canal is common in normal children.

Thus, sagittal widening of the canal in children is not a reliable sign of an expansile intraspinal lesion.

Atlas-dens interval (ADI) in children: A survey based on 200 normal cervical spines. Locke GR, Gardner JI, Van Epps EF, et al. al. *Am J Roentgenol* 1966;97:135-140.
> The atlas-dens interval was measured in 200 normal children 3 to 15 years of age. The tube distance makes a significant difference in evaluating the atlas-dens internal. At a 40-inch tube to film distance there was no measurement greater than 4 mm. At 72 inches, up to 5 mm of atlas-dens internal was identified in normal patients. An excellent anatomical and radiographic description of the upper cervical spine in children is included.

Pseudosubluxation and other normal variations in the cervical spine in children: A study of one hundred and sixty children. Cattell HS, Filtzer DL. *J Bone Joint Surg* 1965;47A:1295-1309.
> This study of 160 normal spine radiographs in children is an excellent description of the radiographic development of the cervical spine and is one of the earliest articles to describe C2-3 pseudosubluxation. Describes the normal ages for the appearance of the basilar odontoid synchondrosis and apical odontoid epiphysis and establishes that cervical lordosis may be absent in normal children.

Hypermobility of the cervical spine in children: A pitfall in the diagnosis of cervical dislocation. Sullivan CR, Bruwer AJ, Harris LE. *Am J Surg* 1958;95:636-640.
> The authors, using roentgenograms from 100 normal children between 2 and 14 years of age, determined the incidence of hypermobility between the second and third and between the third and fourth vertebrae. They determined that this distance can be up to 4 mm in children. Four case reports of cervical spine injuries in children are included.

Tears of the transverse ligament of the atlas: A clinical and biomechanical study. Fielding JW, Cochran GVB, Lawsing JF III, et al. *J Bone Joint Surg* 1974;56A:1683-1691.
> In this biomechanical and clinical study of the strength of the transverse ligament of the atlas, the results of twenty autopsy specimens were correlated with the results in a clinical series of 11 patients with traumatic rupture of the transverse ligament. When tears of the transverse ligament are identified, surgical fusion of C1-2 should be the treatment.

Atlanto-axial instability and spinal cord compression in children: Diagnosis by computerized tomography. Roach JW, Duncan D, Wenger DR, et al. *J Bone Joint Surg* 1984;66A:708-714.
> The computed tomography scan can provide a diagnosis by a non-invasive technique and quantitates the amount of compromise of the spinal cord by delineating flattening of the cord. The scan is helpful in

deciding if the spinal cord is at significant risk and if atlantoaxial fusion is advisable.

Children's cervical spine instability after posterior fossa surgery. Gangemi M, Renier D, Daussange J, et al. *Acta Neurol (Napoli)* 1982;37:39-43.
> The essential factor leading to instability is the number of levels involved. Instability is rare when the lamina of C2 is resected, and increases in frequency when more than 20% of C2 is resected.

The surgical treatment of instability of the upper part of the cervical spine in children and adolescents. Koop SE, Winter RB, Lonstein JE. *J Bone Joint Surg* 1984;66A:403-411.
> Posterior cervical arthrodesis with wire fixation carries some risk of neural injury and often is not applicable in children with anomalous vertebrae. Spine fusion using cautious exposure, delicate decortication by an air-drill, placement of autogenous cancellous iliac grafts, and external immobilization by a halo cast minimizes the risk of neural damage and is a reliable way to obtain a solid arthrodesis.

Observations on the spine in mongoloidism. Martel W, Tishler JM. *Am J Roentgen* 1966;97:630-638.
> This is one of the early articles identifying C1-2 subluxation in Down syndrome. The authors found that six of 37 patients between 2 and 15 years of age, and four of 27 patients between 16 and 32 years of age had abnormal atlanto-dental intervals. This article also describes the abnormalities seen in the thoracic and lumbar spines in these patients. No abnormalities were found in children less than 2 years of age.

Sequelae of atlantoaxial stabilization in two patients with Down's syndrome. Nordt JC, Stauffer ES. *Spine* 1981;6:437-440.
> Two patients developed quadriplegia after manipulative reduction and fusion with sublaminar wiring. Traction is used preoperatively to reduce the deformity and during surgery to maintain alignment. If reduction cannot be obtained, then avoid sublaminar wiring and fuse in situ.

Atlantoaxial instability in individuals with Down syndrome: A fresh look at the evidence. Davidson RG. *Pediatrics* 1988;81:857-865.
> A review of published cases reveals no evidence that current radiographic criteria are predictive of instability. Those who suffered dislocation had preceding neurologic signs for at least several weeks. No atlantoaxial dislocations were reported in 500,000 individuals with Down syndrome while participating in competitive sports.

Atlantoaxial instability in Down syndrome: Roentgenographic, neurologic, and somatosensory evoked potential studies. Pueschel SM, Findley TW, Furia J, et al. *J Pediatr* 1987;110:515-521.
> A combined assessment approach, using roentgenographic, CT scan, neurologic, and neurophysiologic investigations, provides information

about the risk status of patients with Down syndrome and atlantoaxial instability.

Os Odontoideum

Spinal cord compression in Morquio-Brailsford's disease. Blaw ME, Langer LO. *J Pediatr* 1969;74:593-600.
> Eight patients with Morquio's disease had radiographic evidence of hypoplasia or absence of the odontoid as well as thoracic gibbous formation. Reviews spine problems in Morquio's disease, and points out that these should be evaluated before other procedures are performed. Most of the patients had symptomatic neurologic problems with their spinal deformity.

The management of os odontoideum: Analysis of 37 cases. Spierings EL, Braakman R. *J Bone Joint Surg* 1982;64B:422-428.
> Patients with local symptoms should not undergo surgical stabilization unless the space available for the cord is less than 13 mm. Otherwise, they are at significant risk for developing permanent spinal cord injury. Patients with progressive signs or myelopathy should be treated surgically.

Os odontoideum. Fielding JW, Hensinger RN, Hawkins RJ. *J Bone Joint Surg* 1980;62A:376-383.
> Thirty-five patients with os odontoideum were reviewed. Nine patients had a normal odontoid prior to the development of os odontoideum, suggesting a traumatic etiology for this condition. Twenty-two had anterior instability (average 1.03 cm). Five had posterior instability (average 0.84 cm) and 8 had combined instability (average 1.37 cm).

The arterial supply of the odontoid process. Schiff DCM, Parke WW. *J Bone Joint Surg* 1973;55A:1450-1456.
> Detailed description of the blood supply to the odontoid.

Os odontoideum: Clinical, radiological and therapeutic aspects. Minderhoud JM, Braakman R, Penning L. *J Neurol Sci* 1969;8:521-544.
> Five of thirteen patients with os odontoideum presented with progressive myelopathy, four others had transient myelopathy, and the remainder had local cerebral symptoms. Describes the radiographic differences between the congenital and traumatic lesion and establishes that decompressive laminectomy is a highly dangerous procedure that should be avoided in these patients. Surgical fusion should be undertaken despite significant complications. Two deaths and one transient deterioration with surgery occurred in these patients.

The os odontoideum: Separate odontoid process. Wollin DG. *J Bone Joint Surg* 1963;45A:1459-1471.

This article discusses the possibility that os odontoideum is either a lesion created from trauma or a developmental anomaly. Citing several patients with previous injury, the authors postulate that this anomaly may occur secondary to trauma. They present nine cases and state their belief that the patient with an os odontoideum is in less danger of developing neurologic deficit than is the patient with a transverse ligament injury.

CT and myelogram findings of os odontoideum. Teng MM, Shoung HM, Chang CY, et al. *Comput Med Imaging Graph* 1989;13:179-184.

Computed tomographic scan reveals a constriction and/or gap of bony structure between the os odontoideum and the odontoid process. Myelogram showed spinal stenosis as a result of atlantoaxial dislocation or anterior extradural compression from overgrown cartilage and posteriorly dislocated tip of shortened odontoid process. The presence of cartilage may be explained by developmental anomaly or nonunion with pseudarthroses and metaplastic cartilage development.

Klippel-Feil Syndrome

Genitourinary anomalies associated with Klippel-Feil syndrome. Moore WB, Matthews TJ, Rabinowitz R. *J Bone Joint Surg* 1975;57A:355-357.

Of 39 patients with Klippel-Feil syndrome, 25 had significant genitourinary tract anomalies as demonstrated by intravenous pylogram and physical examination. The authors stress that a study of the genitourinary system is part of a routine evaluation of a patient with Klippel-Feil syndrome.

Klippel-Feil syndrome: A constellation of associated anomalies. Hensinger RN, Lang JE, MacEwen GD. *J Bone Joint Surg* 1974;56A:1246-1253.

This is a follow-up of 50 patients with Klippel-Feil syndrome. One third of the patients had renal anomalies, and more than half had scoliosis. Other anomalies found were Sprengel's deformity, impairment of hearing, synkinesia, and congenital heart disease. Patients with Klippel-Keil syndrome should be evaluated for other less apparent anomalies.

Klippel-Feil syndrome. Pizzutillo PD. In Bailey RW (ed): *Cervical Spine.* Philadelphia, JB Lippincott, 1983, pp 174-188.

The best single reference for reviewing Klippel-Feil syndrome. The triad of shortneck, low posterior hairline, and limited range of motion, as well as other clinical findings in Klippel-Feil syndrome, are discussed very thoroughly in this article. History, embryology, associated problems, natural history, and treatment are also described.

Sprengel's Deformity

Congenital elevation of the scapula: Surgical correction by the Woodward procedure. Carson WG, Lovell WW, Whitesides TE Jr. *J Bone Joint Surg* 1981;63A:1199-1207.

> Discusses characteristic findings, associated congenital anomalies, indications for operation, and surgical techniques. Stresses the importance of the rotational component of Sprengel's deformity.

Congenital elevation of the scapula: Correction by release and transplantation of muscle origins. A preliminary report. Woodward JW. *J Bone Joint Surg* 1961;43A:219-228.

> This original description of Woodward's surgical procedure to correct congenital elevation of the scapula is illustrated with drawings and describes the results in nine patients. There was improvement in cosmesis with no improvement in shoulder function. One patient had brachial palsy develop following the correction.

Sprengel deformity. Leibovic SJ, Ehrlich MG, Zaleske DJ. *J Bone Joint Surg* 1990;72A:192-197.

> This is a review of 15 cases of Sprengel deformity. In 11 of the 15, there was moderate or dramatic improvement in cosmetic appearance. The original malrotation of the scapula, corrected initially, usually recurred after about two years. Describes a useful radiographic method to quantitate lowering and derotation of the scapula.

Torticollis

Congenital muscular torticollis in infancy: Some observations regarding treatment. Coventry MB, Harris LE. *J Bone Joint Surg* 1959;41A:815-822.

> This excellent classic review of 35 patients with congenital muscular torticollis presents physical and pathological findings, treatment, and follow-up.

Sternomastoid tumour and muscular torticollis. Macdonald D. *J Bone Joint Surg* 1969;51B:432-443.

> Evaluates the relationship between the sternomastoid tumor and congenital muscular torticollis. It reviews the etiology and pathogenesis of the condition and presents 152 children with torticollis.

Idiopathic torticollis: Sternocleidomastoid myopathy and accessory neuropathy. Sarnat HB, Morrissy RT. *Muscle Nerve* 1981;4:374-380.

> The unique blood supply to the sternal head of the muscle predisposes it to ischemia, resulting in focal myopathy and fibrosis. The clavicular head demonstrates progressive denervation caused by entrapment of the accessory nerve as it traverses the sternal head, which results in further deformity.

Muscular torticollis: Late results of operative treatment. Staheli LT. *Surgery* 1971;69:469-473.

> This is a long-term follow-up of 14 patients treated for congenital muscular torticollis. At follow-up patients had few complaints. A tight recurrent lateral band was evident in five patients, and two patients had a second release. In this study, early operation did not appear to reduce the likelihood of late residual facial asymmetry.

Congenital muscular torticollis: A long-term follow-up. Canale ST, Griffin DW, Hubbard CN. *J Bone Joint Surg* 1982;64A:810-816.

> If this condition persists beyond one year of age, it does not resolve spontaneously, and nonsurgical therapy is rarely successful. Established facial asymmetry and limitation of motion of more than 30 degrees usually precludes a good result.

The influence of age on the results of open sternomastoid tenotomy in muscular torticollis. Ling CM. *Clin Orthop* 1976;116:142-148.

> This is a report of 60 patients who underwent sternocleidomastoid release for congenital muscular torticollis. They found the best time for surgery in this condition is between 1 and 4 years of age. There were complications with scarring in patients less than 1 year old as well as in those over 5. Overall the results were very acceptable in all age groups.

Muscular torticollis: A modified surgical approach. Ferkel RD, Westin GW, Dawson EG, et al. *J Bone Joint Surg* 1983;65A:894-900.

> Twelve children were treated by a modified bipolar release of the sternocleidomastoid muscle. The muscle is released at the mastoid process and at its clavicular insertion. The sternal insertion is retained but is lengthened by a Z-plasty. The modified bipolar release had a greater percentage of good or excellent results than were seen in ten patients who underwent other surgical procedures.

The coexistence of torticollis and congenital dysplasia of the hip. Hummer CD Jr, MacEwen GD. *J Bone Joint Surg* 1972;54A:1255-1256.

> This is a brief report of a ten-year study of children with torticollis. It was found that 20% of the children with torticollis had either congenital hip dislocation or subluxation. Recommends that all children with congenital muscular torticollis undergo a careful clinical and possible radiographic examination of the hip.

Gastroesophageal reflux and torticollis. Ramenofsky ML, Buyse M, Goldberg MJ, et al. *J Bone Joint Surg* 1978;60A:1140-1141.

> Sandifer's syndrome is a combination of hiatal hernia and abnormal posturing of the head and neck. The abnormal posturing has been attributed to an attempt to decrease the pain of esophagitis resulting from gastroesophageal reflux and hiatal hernia.

Torticollis in children caused by congenital anomalies of the atlas. Dubousset J. *J Bone Joint Surg* 1986;68A:178-188.

Congenital hypoplasia of the atlas may result in severe and progressive torticollis. Abnormality of the vertebral arteries is common. Observation is indicated except in the presence of severe torticollis or of instability, in which case surgical fusion becomes the appropriate treatment.

Intervertebral disc calcification syndromes in children. Sonnabend DH, Taylor TK, Chapman GK. *J Bone Joint Surg* 1982;64B:25-31.
Cervical involvement is most common. There is an abrupt onset of symptoms; pain in the neck, torticollis, and reduced range of motion. Neurologic symptoms are rare. Rapid clinical and gradual radiographic resolution is expected.

Atlanto-axial rotatory fixation (fixed rotatory subluxation of the atlantoaxial joint). Fielding JW, Hawkins RJ. *J Bone Joint Surg* 1977;59A:37-44.
Reports 17 cases of fixed rotatory fixation of C1 and C2. This study included seven children, all of whom presented late and had fixed, often unreducible, subluxation. Describes the treatment, including skull traction and atlantoaxial arthrodesis, if necessary.

The management of rotatory atlanto-axial subluxation in children. Phillips WA, Hensinger RN. *J Bone Joint Surg* 1989;71A:664-668.
Rotatory atlantoaxial subluxation was reviewed in 23 children. If symptoms had persisted less than a month, the subluxation reduced either spontaneously or after a brief period of traction. Three of the seven were seen more than a month after the onset of symptoms and required C1-C2 arthrodesis. Dynamic computed tomographic scans proved the most satisfactory method of documenting this condition.

Vertebral Column

Stuart L. Weinstein, MD

Adolescent Idiopathic Scoliosis

Moe's Textbook of Scoliosis and Other Spinal Deformities, ed 2. In Bradford DS, Lonstein JE, Moe JH, et al (eds). Philadelphia, WB Saunders, 1987.
> This classic textbook on all aspects of scoliosis has an extensive bibliography, and is well illustrated.

Adolescent idiopathic scoliosis. Screening and diagnosis, Lonstein JE, pp 105-113. Adolescent idiopathic scoliosis: Prevalence and natural history, Weinstein SL, pp 115-128. Nonoperative treatment of adolescent idiopathic scoliosis, Keller RB, pp 129-135. Preoperative and intraoperative considerations in adolescent idiopathic scoliosis, Engler GL, pp 137-141. Surgical treatment of adolescent idiopathic scoliosis, Tolo VT, pp 243-256. In Barr JS (ed): American Academy of Orthopaedic Surgeons *Instructional Course Lectures, XXXVIII*. Park Ridge, IL, American Academy of Orthopaedic Surgeons, 1989, pp 105-156.
> These chapters cover screening, diagnosis, prevalence, natural history, nonoperative treatment, pre- and intraoperative considerations, and surgical management of adolescent idiopathic scoliosis.

Scoliosis. Winter RB (ed). *Orthop Clin North Am* 1988;19:227-465.
> Brief monograph covering aspects of scoliosis of varying etiologies.

Prevalence and Natural History

Natural history of untreated idiopathic scoliosis after skeletal maturity. Ascani E, Bartolozzi P, Logroscino CA, et al. *Spine* 1986;11:784-789.
> Multicenter average 34-year follow-up of 187 untreated idiopathic scoliosis patients. The authors address incidence and factors related to pulmonary function, pain, psychosocial effects, and curve progression.

Idiopathic scoliosis: Natural History. Weinstein SL. *Spine* 1986;11:780-783.
> Review of 54 patients with complete radiographs from initial presentation through skeletal maturity, 30-year and 40-year follow-up. Radiographic factors leading to curve progression at maturity also apply to skeletally immature patients.

The prediction of curve progression in untreated idiopathic scoliosis during growth. Lonstein JE, Carlson JM. *J Bone Joint Surg* 1984;66A:1061-1071.

The risk of progression is studied in 727 patients. A curve of 20 degrees to 29 degrees in a Risser 0-1 patient has a 68% chance of progression, while a curve less than 20 degrees in a Risser 2-4 patient has only 1.6% of progression. Other risk factors in progression are discussed.

The natural history of idiopathic scoliosis before skeletal maturity. Bunnell WP. *Spine* 1986;11:773-776.
This study of 326 patients assesses the risk factors in progression.

Curve progression in idiopathic scoliosis. Weinstein SL, Ponseti IV. *J Bone Joint Surg* 1983;65A:477-455.
After skeletal maturity, 68% of curves progressed. Presents factors leading to curve progression after maturity.

Incidence and severity of back pain in adult idiopathic scoliosis. Jackson RP, Simmons EH, Stripinis D. *Spine* 1983;8:749-756.
Adults with idiopathic scoliosis (197) are compared with a control group of 180 adults without spinal deformity, as regards back pain (equal in both groups) and the clinical course of back pain.

Scoliosis in the elderly: A follow-up study. Robin GC, Span Y, Steinberg R, et al. *Spine* 1982;7:355-359.
Scoliosis of a minor degree is very common in the elderly, many curves arising de novo. Curves do progress in the elderly. There is no relationship between scoliosis and osteoporosis, back pain, or degenerative changes in the spine.

Idiopathic scoliosis: Long-term follow-up and prognosis in untreated patients. Weinstein SL, Zavala DC, Ponseti IV. *J Bone Joint Surg* 1981;63A:702-712.
Patients with untreated adolescent idiopathic scoliosis (194) are reviewed with a follow-up of 39.3 years. Incidence of backache was slightly less than in the general population. In some patients, progression occurred during adulthood, especially in thoracic curves that measured between 50 and 80 degrees at the end of growth. Pulmonary function, psychosocial effects, mortality, and morbidity are discussed.

The incidence of low-back pain in adult scoliosis. Kostuik JP, Bentivoglio J. *Spine* 1981;6:268-273.
A review of IVPs in 5,000 patients (the majority in the sixth to eighth decades) shows a 3.9% incidence of lumbar curves over 10 degrees. Of the 5,000, 59% had back pain, about the same as in the general population. Pain was more common in patients with facet sclerosis (not osteophytes) and was more severe in patients with curves over 45 degrees.

Adult scoliosis and back pain. Nachemson A. *Spine* 1979;4:513-517.
Surgery for scoliosis in the adult is unusual. Some curves arise de novo in the adult due to disc degeneration and osteoporosis. The incidence of

back pain in adults with scoliosis is no different from that in adults with straight spines.

Scoliosis: Incidence and natural history: A prospective epidemiological study. Rogala EJ, Drummond DS, Gurr J. *J Bone Joint Surg* 1978;60A:173-176.
> Prospective study on incidence and early natural history regarding curve progression. Based on a screened population of 26,947 children.

School Screening

Symposium on school screening for scoliosis: Scoliosis Research Society and British Scoliosis Society, Ashworth, MA (ed). *Spine* 1988;13:1177-1200.
> This excellent series of papers defines the screening process and evaluates results to date. Pros and cons of school screening are effectively discussed.

Voluntary school screening for scoliosis in Minnesota. Lonstein JE, Bjorklund S, Wanninger MH, et al. *J Bone Joint Surg* 1982;64A:481-488.
> Of 250,000 children examined each year, 3.4% were referred for evaluation and 1.2% were found to have scoliosis. Screening has markedly decreased the number of patients needing surgery.

A prospective prevalence study of scoliosis in Southern Sweden. Willner S, Udén A. *Acta Orthop Scand* 1982;53:233-237.
> Prospective prevalence study of 17,181 children born in Malmo between 1961 and 1965 and screened from 1971 to 1980. Gives breakdown by sex, curve pattern, progression, and need for treatment.

The changing pattern of scoliosis treatment due to effective screening. Torell G, Nordwall A, Nachemson A. *J Bone Joint Surg* 1981;63A:337-341.
> A ten-year program was evaluated. A three-fold increase in the number of patients treated is noted, with a significant decrease in the curve severity at diagnosis. Because of the early diagnosis, most patients needing treatment do not require surgery.

Etiology

Pathogenesis of idiopathic scoliosis: Proceedings of an International Conference. Jacobs RR, (ed). Scoliosis Research Society, Chicago, IL, 1984.
> Multiauthor monograph from a symposium on pathogenesis of scoliosis at the Scoliosis Research Society. Good compilation of articles on all etiologic theories for idiopathic scoliosis.

Idiopathic scoliosis and the central nervous system: A motor control problem. The Harrington lecture, 1983. Scoliosis Research Society. Herman R, Mixon J, Fisher A, et al. *Spine* 1985;10:1-14.

45

Proposes an etiologic concept linking an impaired axial motor control system to the structural deformity of idiopathic scoliosis.

The pathogenesis of idiopathic scoliosis: Biplanar spinal asymmetry. Dickson RA, Lawton JO, Archer IA, et al. *J Bone Joint Surg* 1984;66B:8-15.
Presents evidence that when flattening or reversal of normal thoracic kyphosis at the apex of a scoliosis is superimposed during growth, a progressive idiopathic scoliosis results. Includes clinical, cadaveric, biomechanical, and radiological material supporting this theory.

Etiologic factors in adolescent idiopathic scoliosis. Nachemson AL, Sahlstrand T. *Spine* 1977;2:176-184.
Summary of various etiologic theories of idiopathic scoliosis.

Nonsurgical Treatment

Electrical stimulation in the treatment of idiopathic scoliosis. O'Donnell CS, Bunnell WP, Betz RR, et al. *Clin Orthop* 1988;229:107-113.
Report of 62 patients treated with an electrospinal orthosis and evaluated at average 2.3-year follow-up. Curve progression exceeds the expected risk of curve progression of untreated curves. The results demonstrate that electrical stimulation fails to alter the natural history of idiopathic scoliosis.

Further evaluation of the Scolitron treatment of idiopathic adolescent scoliosis. Sullivan JA, Davidson R, Renshaw TS, et al. *Spine* 1986;11:903-906.
Review of 142 patients treated by lateral electrical surface stimulation. Reports 26.8% success and 56.3% failure rates. Patients at risk for progression had the highest failure rates.

The effectiveness of bracing in the nonoperative treatment of idiopathic scoliosis. Winter RB, Lonstein JE, Drogt J, et al. *Spine* 1986;11:790-791.
Reviews 95 high-risk patents with thoracic curves treated by Milwaukee Brace (23 hours/day with slow weaning at Risser 4). Average follow-up was 2.5 years out of brace or until surgery. Brace halted progression in 84% of cases.

Part-time bracing of adolescent idiopathic scoliosis. Green NE. *J Bone Joint Surg* 1986;68A:738-742.
Fifty-five month average follow-up of 44 skeletally immature patients treated by 16 hours per day of brace wear. The author reports improved compliance and demonstrated that this program can prevent curve progression.

Effectiveness of braces in mild idiopathic scoliosis. Miller JA, Nachemson AL, Schultz AB. *Spine* 1984;9:632-635.
Follow-up for a mean period of 1.9 years of two comparable groups, one treated with Milwaukee or Boston Brace and the other untreated.

Bracing reduced the probability of progression (not statistically significant). Study points out the problems with most brace studies and suggests need for controlled, randomized, prospective study of brace effectiveness (currently underway under auspices of Scoliosis Research Society).

Multicenter trial of a noninvasive stimulation method for idiopathic scoliosis: A summary of early treatment results. Brown JC, Axelgaard J, Howson DC. *Spine* 1984;9:382-387.
Results of multicenter trial with lateral surface electrical stimulation.

Radiation hazards in scoliosis management. Drummond D, Ranallo F, Lonstein J, et al. *Spine* 1983;8:741-748.
Reviews risks of radiation in diagnosis and management of scoliosis. Gives recommendations for reducing radiation risks while obtaining necessary diagnostic information.

Miami thoracolumbosacral orthosis in the management of scoliosis: Preliminary results in 100 cases. McCollough NC III, Schultz M, Javech N, et al. *J Pediatr Orthop* 1981;1:141-152.
Preliminary results of underarm bracing for scoliosis in 100 patients.

Treatment of idiopathic scoliosis in the Milwaukee Brace. Carr WA, Moe JH, Winter RB, et al. *J Bone Joint Surg* 1980;62A:599-612.
Results of 74 patients are analyzed 5 years or more after brace removal. No patient required surgery, but 80% showed some curve progression. Curves over 40 degrees did less well than curves under 40 degrees. Curves showing a good initial response to the brace did better.

Current concepts review: Scoliosis bracing. Nash CL Jr. *J Bone Joint Surg* 1980;62A:848-852.
Summarizes concepts, principles, and materials used in scoliosis bracing.

Modern concepts of treatment of spinal deformities in children and adults. Moe JH. *Clin Orthop* 1980;150:137-153.
Summary article on treatment principles of scoliosis, including bracing and surgery.

The effect of an exercise program on change in curve in adolescents with minimal idiopathic scoliosis: A preliminary study. Stone B, Beekman C, Hall V, et al. *Phys Ther* 1979;59:759-763.
Controlled study of the effectiveness of an exercise program. Treated patients did no better than untreated patients.

Surgical Treatment

Surgical treatment of adolescent idiopathic scoliosis: A comparative analysis.
Mielke CH, Lonstein JE, Denis F, et al. *J Bone Joint Surg* 1989;71A:1170-
1177.
>   Detailed review of 352 patients with single right or double thoracic
>   curves who underwent posterior arthrodesis plus one of four different
>   instrumentation systems--Harrington distraction rod, Harrington
>   distraction plus compression rod, Harrington distraction plus
>   compression rods and a device for transverse traction, and Harrington
>   distraction rod with sublaminar wires. The authors demonstrated
>   satisfactory results with each system and outline the indication for each
>   depending on the anteroposterior and sagittal plane deformity.
>   Immobilization after surgery was a critical factor in maintaining
>   correction.

Frontal plane and sagittal plane balance following Cotrel-Dubousset
instrumentation for idiopathic scoliosis. Richards BS, Birch JG, Herring JA, et
al. *Spine* 1989;14:733-737.
>   Authors evaluated frontal and sagittal plane balance in 53 patients to
>   determine optimum levels for fusion. Paper is one of several pointing
>   out problems with postoperative decompensation using the Cotrel-
>   Dubousset instrumentation and demonstrating that the rules outlined by
>   King and associates for selecting the fusion area may not apply using
>   Cotrel-Dubousset instrumentation.

Adult idiopathic scoliosis treated with Luque or Harrington rods and sublaminar
wiring. Winter RB, Lonstein JE. *J Bone Joint Surg* 1989;71A:1308-1313.
>   Average three-year follow-up report of 42 adults with adolescent
>   idiopathic scoliosis treated by posterior fusion and sublaminar wires
>   attached to Harrington or double-L-shaped Luque rods. Thirteen
>   patients had preliminary anterior arthrodesis. Surgery was
>   uncomplicated in 71%. Pseudoarthrosis was seen in 7% of the series
>   but in 13% of those having posterior arthrodesis alone. One neurologic
>   complication was reported. The effect of the operation on pain,
>   pulmonary function, or cosmesis was not studied.

Spinous process segmental instrumentation for scoliosis. Herzenberg JE,
Coonrad RW, Ross DB, et al. *J Spinal Disorders* 1988;1:206-210.
>   Reviews 75 cases (61 with idiopathic scoliosis) using this technique.
>   Authors conclude that spinous process segmental instrumentation is an
>   effective alternative to Harrington instrumentation or Luque sublaminar
>   segmental instrumentation and avoids the increased neurologic risk
>   associated with passage of sublaminar wires or the need for
>   postoperative casting.

New universal instrumentation in spinal surgery. Cotrel Y, Dubousset J,
Guillaumat M. *Clin Orthop* 1988;227:10-23.

Describes instrumentation and principles of application of this system to address the three-dimensional aspects of spinal deformity. The authors present preliminary results in 250 patients.

Results of surgical treatment of adults with idiopathic scoliosis. Sponseller PD, Cohen MS, Nachemson AL, et al. *J Bone Joint Surg* 1987;69A:667-675.
Follow-up (7.3-year average) of 45 patients surgically treated as adults for scoliosis. Peak and constant pain levels decreased but frequency of peak pain after surgery was unchanged. Functional impairment was lessened, but pulmonary function remained unchanged. Forty percent had a minor complication and 20% had a major complication.

Adolescent idiopathic scoliosis treated by Harrington rod distraction and fusion. Lovallo JL, Banta JV, Renshaw TS. *J Bone Joint Surg* 1986;68A:1326-1330.
In a 44-month mean follow-up of 133 surgically treated patients, the authors demonstrated that a single Harrington distraction rod and fusion, followed by 6 months in a postoperative cast, is a safe and effective treatment for adolescent idiopathic scoliosis. There were no neurologic injuries.

Interspinous process segmental spinal instrumentation. Drummond D, Guadagni J, Keene JS, et al. *J Pediatr Orthop* 1984;4:397-404.
Technique, laboratory testing, and early clinical results are described for a method of interspinous segmental spinal instrumentation (ISSI). Method avoids risks associated with passage of sublaminar wires.

The selection of fusion levels in thoracic idiopathic scoliosis. King HA, Moe JH, Bradford DS, et al. *J Bone Joint Surg* 1983;65A:1302-1313.
Analyzes 405 patients as to the proper selection of fusion levels. Discusses issue of when to fuse a lumbar curve.

Long-term follow-up of scoliosis fusion. Moskowitz A, Moe JH, Winter RB, et al. *J Bone Joint Surg* 1980;62A:364-376.
Sixty-one patients reviewed after an average follow-up of 26 years following posterior spinal fusion show stable fusions with low back pain not a significant problem.

An eleven-year clinical investigation of Harrington instrumentation: A preliminary report on 578 cases. Harrington PR, Dickson JH. *Clin Orthop* 1973;93:113-130.
Historical overview of the development of Harrington instrumentation, fusion technique and post-operative regime. Presents results of various groups of patients treated during the evolution of techniques and management.

Spinal Cord Monitoring

Current concepts review: Spinal cord monitoring. Nash CL Jr, Brown RH. *J Bone Joint Surg* 1989;71A:627-630.
>This review article outlines the various types of spinal cord monitoring currently in use and gives their advantages and disadvantages.

Juvenile Idiopathic Scoliosis

Juvenile idiopathic scoliosis. Figueiredo UM, James JI. *J Bone Joint Surg* 1981;63B:61-66.
>Review of 98 patients with juvenile idiopathic scoliosis. Curve patterns are analyzed and results of treatment by observation, bracing, and surgery are presented.

The characteristics of juvenile idiopathic scoliosis and results of its treatment. Tolo VT, Gillespie R. *J Bone Joint Surg* 1978;60B:181-188.
>Review of 59 patients with juvenile idiopathic scoliosis. The prognostic value of the rib vertebral angle difference is discussed.

Infantile Idiopathic Scoliosis

Prognosis in infantile idiopathic scoliosis. Ceballos T, Ferrer-Torrelles M, Castillo F, et al. *J Bone Joint Surg* 1980;62A:863-875.
>Reviews 113 patients with infantile scoliosis, giving prognosis relative to sex, age at onset, and Mehta angle. Confirms Mehta's prognostic criteria.

The non-operative treatment of infantile idiopathic scoliosis. Mehta MH, Morel G. In Zorab PA, Siegler D (eds): *Scoliosis*. Academic Press, London, 1980, pp 71-84.
>Summary article in the approach to the patient with infantile scoliosis and the results of nonsurgical treatment.

Congenital Scoliosis and Kyphosis

Congenital Deformities of the Spine. Winter RB (ed). New York, Thieme-Stratton, 1983.
>This overview of congenital spine deformities is based on the author's extensive experience.

Hemivertebra as a cause of scoliosis: A study of 104 patients. McMaster MJ, David CV. *J Bone Joint Surg* 1986;68B:588-595.
>Review of natural history of 154 hemivertebrae (65% fully segmented, nonincarcerated; 22% semisegmented, and 12% incarcerated) in 104 patients. Risk factors include type of hemivertebrae, location, age of

patient, and number of hemivertebrae and their relationship to each other. Fully segmented, nonincarcerated hemivertebrae may require prophylactic treatment to prevent significant deformity: semisegmented and incarcerated hemivertebrae usually require no treatment.

Occult intraspinal anomalies and congenital scoliosis. McMaster MJ. *J Bone Joint Surg* 1984;66A:588-601.
> Excellent review of incidence and pathology of occult intraspinal congenital abnormalities associated with congenital scoliosis. Of the 251 patients in this series, 18% had occult intraspinal abnormalities. Diastematomyelia was the most common lesion and was most commonly associated with unilateral unsegmented bars with contralateral hemivertebrae in the lower thoracic or thoracolumbar region.

Natural History

Congenital scoliosis: A study of 234 patients treated and untreated. Part I: Natural history. Part II: Treatment. Winter RB, Moe JH, Eilers VE. *J Bone Joint Surg* 1968;50A:15-47.
> Natural history and treatment study of a large group of patients with congenital scoliosis. Indications for treatment are based on natural history of pathologic lesion and its location in the spine.

Progression of congenital scoliosis due to hemivertebrae and hemivertebrae with bars. Nasco RJ, Stilling FH III, Stell HH. *J Bone Joint Surg* 1975;57A:456-466.
> The authors classify 60 cases of congenital scoliosis and kyphoscoliosis due to hemivertebrae or unilateral bar associated with hemivertebrae into 6 types. Prognostic factors include location of hemivertebrae and presence of unilateral bars. Rates of progression are discussed.

The natural history of congenital scoliosis: A study of two hundred and fifty-one patients. McMaster MJ, Ohtsuka K. *J Bone Joint Surg* 1982;64A:1128-1147.
> Review of natural history of 251 patients with congenital scoliosis. Abnormalities are classified as regards prognosis for each pattern and curve location.

Etiology

Congenital kyphosis by segmentation defect: Etiologic and pathogenic studies. Morin B, Poitras B, Duhaime M, et al. *J Pediatr Orthop* 1985;5:309-314.
> Presents clinical and research evidence to support the theory that kyphosis resulting from segmentation defect represents a developmental defect of the perivertebral structures, including the annulus fibrosus, the ring apophysis, and anterior longitudinal ligament, rather than an intervertebral bar.

Embryogenesis and prenatal development of congenital vertebral anomalies and their classification. Tsou PM, Yau A, Hodgson AR. *Clin Orthop* 1980;152:211-231.

>   Reviews anomalies in 144 patients and evaluates 15 embryos and fetuses. Classification of anomalies is based on specific defects, pathogenesis, and time of origin in embryonic or fetal development.

Congenital vertebral malformations: Time of induction in human and mouse embryo. Rivard CH, Narbaitz R, Uhthoff HK. *Orthop Rev* 1979;8:135-139.

>   Presents experimental evidence for role of hypoxia in etiology of congenital spine deformities.

Development of the vertebral column as related to certain congenital and pathological changes. Ehrenhaft JL. *Surg Gynecol Obstetr* 1943;76:282-292.

>   Classic embryologic study on spine development.

Treatment

Convex growth arrest for progressive congenital scoliosis due to hemivertebrae. Winter RB, Lonstein JE, Denis F, et al. *J Pediatr Orthop* 1988;8:633-638.

>   Follow-up (6.5 years) of convex anteroposterior hemiarthrodesis, hemiepiphysiodesis in 13 patients with progressive congenital scoliosis due to hemivertebrae or hemivertebrae associated with other spinal anomalies. Progression was arrested in 12 of 13, and five of the 12 showed progressive improvement. Surgical technique and patient selection criteria are described.

The surgical treatment of congenital kyphosis: A review of 94 patients age 5 years or older, with 2 years or more follow-up in 77 patients. Winter RB, Moe JH, Lonstein JE. *Spine* 1985;10:224-231.

>   Seven-year average follow-up of 94 patients with congenital kyphosis (27 were treated by posterior fusion alone; 48 were treated by combined anterior and posterior fusion). Curve correction and maintenance was better in the combined group. Pseudarthrosis occurred in 31% of the patients treated only by posterior fusions compared with 8% of the combined group. Posterior fusion alone may have limited value in children and adolescents with kyphosis less than 55 degrees.

Posterior spinal arthrodesis for congenital scoliosis: An analysis of the cases of two hundred and ninety patients, five to nineteen years old. Winter RB, Moe JH, Lonstein JE. *J Bone Joint Surg* 1984;66A:1188-1197.

>   Six-year follow-up of 290 patients treated between the ages of 5 and 19 years by posterior spinal arthrodesis, with or without Harrington instrumentation. The most common problem, bending of the fusion mass, occurred in 40 patients (14%). Use of distraction instrumentation gave only slightly better correction but was associated with the only case of paraplegia. Bending of the fusion is probably a function of growth discrepancy between the concave and convex sides.

The results of spinal arthrodesis for congenital spinal deformity in patients younger than five years old. Winter RB, Moe JH. *J Bone Joint Surg* 1982;64A:419-432.

> This follow-up review of 49 patients treated surgically at less than 5 years of age outlines the role for early posterior fusion.

Surgical treatment of congenital scoliosis with or without Harrington instrumentation. Hall JE, Herndon WA, Levine CR. *J Bone Joint Surg* 1981;63A:608-619.

> Reviews surgical management of 31 patients with congenital scoliosis. Covers pre-operative evaluation, recommendation, and choice of technique.

Congenital kyphosis due to defects of anterior segmentation. Mayfield JK, Winter RB, Bradford DS, et al. *J Bone Joint Surg* 1980;62A:1291-1301.

> Reviews 27 patients with Type II congenital kyphosis. Milwaukee brace has little effect. Early recognition and posterior fusion are recommended.

Congenital kyphosis: Its natural history and treatment as observed in a study of one hundred and thirty patients. Winter RB, Moe JH, Wang JF. *J Bone Joint Surg* 1973;55A:223-256.

> Defines the three types of congenital kyphosis and reports the results of natural history, bracing, and surgical intervention. Presents surgical techniques and treatment indications.

Scheuermann's Disease and Postural Roundback

Reciprocal angulation of vertebral bodies in a sagittal plane: Approach to references for the evaluation of kyphosis and lordosis. Stagnara P, De Mauroy JC, Dran G, et al. *Spine* 1982;7:335-342.

> Discusses values, based on radiographs in 100 patients, of normal thoracic kyphosis and lumbar lordosis.

Juvenile kyphosis: An ultrastructural study. Ippolito E, Bellocci M, Montanaro A, et al. *J Pediatr Orthop* 1985;5:315-322.

> Presents histologic and histochemical studies of the intervertebral disc, vertebral plate, growth plate, and part of the vertebral body in seven patients. The paper confirms previously presented findings based on a single case.

Juvenile kyphosis: Histological and histochemical studies. Ippolito E, Ponseti IV. *J Bone Joint Surg* 1981;63A:175-182.

> The pathology and histology of Scheuermann's disease are presented and compared to normal. Etiology is discussed based on the pathologic findings.

Scheuermann kyphosis: Follow-up of Milwaukee-brace treatment. Sachs B, Bradford D, Winter R, et al. *J Bone Joint Surg* 1987;69A:50-57.

> In this long-term follow-up (five years or more) of 120 patients treated for Scheuermann's disease with a Milwaukee brace, the authors found the Milwaukee brace to be an effective method of treatment for patients with Scheuermann's kyphosis, with 69% of patients showing improvement. However, those with an initial kyphosis of more than 74 degrees had a higher percentage of unsatisfactory results.

Scheuermann's kyphosis: Long-term results of Milwaukee braces treatment. Montgomery SP, Erwin WE. *Spine* 1981;6:5-8.

> Correction of curvature is demonstrated in this follow-up study of 39 patients. However, later follow-up, at 15 months out of brace, shows relapse, indicating that lasting results require brace treatment for longer than 18 months.

Scheuermann's kyphosis and roundback deformity: Results of Milwaukee brace treatment. Bradford DS, Moe JH, Montalvo FJ, et al. *J Bone Joint Surg* 1974;56A:740-758.

> Reports results of Milwaukee brace treatment in 223 patients. Factors influencing Milwaukee bracing results are presented.

Surgical management of thoracic kyphosis in adolescents. Taylor TC, Wenger DR, Stephen J, et al. *J Bone Joint Surg* 1979;61A:496-503.

> Reports results of surgery and short-term follow-up of 27 patients treated for Scheuermann's disease or juvenile round back.

The surgical management of patients with Scheuermann's disease: A review of twenty-four cases managed by combined anterior and posterior spine fusion. Bradford DS, Ahmed KB, Moe JH, et al. *J Bone Joint Surg* 1980;62A:705-712.

> Results of combined anterior and posterior surgery are reported in 24 patients: Complications and pitfalls in treatment are discussed.

Lumbar Scheuermann's: A clinical series and classification. Blumenthal SL, Roach J, Herring JA. *Spine* 1987;12:929-932.

> The authors present 13 cases of lumbar Scheuermann's disease (T10-L4). Six patients had classic changes (Sorenson criteria) with only one having back pain. Six patients had typical changes of end plate irregularity, anterior Schmorl's node, and disc space narrowing, and all had back pain. Based on these findings, the authors propose a new classification for lumbar Scheuermann's disease.

Miscellaneous Spine Deformities

Cerebral Palsy and Neuromuscular Scoliosis

Spinal fusion augmented by Luque-rod segmental instrumentation for neuromuscular scoliosis. Broom MJ, Banta JV, Renshaw TS. *J Bone Joint Surg* 1989;71A:32-44.

> Although fewer than half of the patients in the series had cerebral palsy, this diagnosis accounted for the largest group in the paper. With a mean follow-up of 42 months, the authors demonstrate that Luque-rod segmental instrumentation with posterior spinal instrumentation is an effective treatment for patients with neuromuscular scoliosis. Failure rates were higher when the smaller, 3/16th-inch rods were used, and functional kyphosis occurred above the fusion when it did not extend to the upper thoracic spine.

Management of neuromuscular spinal deformities with Luque segmental instrumentation. Boachie-Adjei O, Lonstein JE, Winter RB, et al. *J Bone Joint Surg* 1989;71A:548-562.

> Average three-year follow-up of 46 patients with neuromuscular scoliosis. Of the 46 patients, 22 (48%) had cerebral palsy. The authors discuss the indication for surgery, need for pelvic extension of the instrumentation and fusion, role of postoperative immobilization, role of two-stage procedures, and complications in this most difficult group of patients.

Considerations in the treatment of cerebral palsy patients with spinal deformities. Ferguson RL, Allen BL Jr. *Orthop Clin North Am* 1988;19:419-425.

> This review article covers all aspects of decision making with regard to spinal deformity in patients with cerebral palsy.

The treatment of scoliosis in cerebral palsy by posterior spinal fusion with Luque-rod segmental instrumentation. Gersoff WK, Renshaw TS. *J Bone Joint Surg* 1988;70A:41-44.

> Review of 33 patients with cerebral palsy who underwent posterior spinal fusion and Luque-rod instrumentation at a mean follow-up of 40 months. Luque rodding accompanying posterior spinal fusion allows safe correction of the deformity, maintenance of correction, and achievement of a solid spinal fusion with minimal complications.

Operative treatment of spinal deformities in patients with cerebral palsy or mental retardation: An analysis of one hundred and seven cases. Lonstein JE, Akbarnia A. *J Bone Joint Surg* 1983;65A:43-55.

> Follow-up of 107 cases at 4.5 years. Presents evaluation of techniques and approach to patients. Makes recommendations concerning timing and techniques of surgery, and reviews complications.

Neuromuscular spine deformities. Lonstein JE, Renshaw TS. In Griffin PP (ed): American Academy of Orthopaedic Surgeons *Instructional Course Lectures, XXXVI*. Park Ridge, IL, American Academy of Orthopaedic Surgeons, 1987, pp 285-304.

> A good review of the etiology, characteristics, orthotic and seating device options, surgical principles, and techniques for neuromuscular spine deformities. The section on cerebral palsy is particularly extensive and reflects the authors' experience and research.

Myelomeningocele

Scoliosis in myelomeningocele. Samuelsson L, Eklof O. *Acta Orthop Scand* 1988;59:122-127.

> Reviews the prevalence, type, and magnitude of scoliosis in 163 patients with myelomeningocele. Of these patients, 143 developed scoliosis, of which 15% were congenital in origin. Scoliosis severity increased with higher neurologic level (particularly above L3) and increasing age. Curve direction correlated with pelvic obliquity, but not with hip dislocation.

Anterior and posterior instrumentation and fusion of thoracolumbar scoliosis due to myelomeningocele. McMaster MJ. *J Bone Joint Surg* 1987;69B:20-25.

> The author demonstrates improved posture and function in 21 of 23 patients with myelomeningocele scoliosis treated by anterior and posterior spinal instrumentation and fusion. Discusses indications, operative techniques, and complications.

Efficacy of surgical management for scoliosis in myelomeningocele: Correction of deformity and alteration of functional status. Mazur J, Menelaus MB, Dickens DR, et al. *J Pediatr Orthop* 1986;6:568-575.

> The authors evaluated the effect of spinal fusion in 49 patients with myelomeningocele. Combined anterior interbody fusion and posterior fusion and instrumentation to the sacrum gave the best correction of the deformity. The ability to ambulate, however, was adversely affected.

Surgical treatment of paralytic scoliosis associated with myelomeningocele. Osebold WR, Mayfield JK, Winter RB, et al. *J Bone Joint Surg* 1982;64A:841-856.

> Discusses results and evolution of treatment of scoliosis in meningomyelocele.

Scoliosis and hydrocephalus in myelocele patients: The effects of ventricular shunting. Hall P, Lindseth R, Campbell R, et al. *J Neurosurg* 1979;50:174-178.

> Progressive scoliosis may be due to shunt malfunction. The importance of neurologic exams at each visit is stressed.

Vertebral excision for kyphosis in children with myelomeningocele. Lindseth RE, Stelzer L Jr. *J Bone Joint Surg* 1979;61A:699-704.

> Presents a method of kyphectomy that allows continued growth of the remaining lumbar spine.

Management of myelomeningocele kyphosis in the older child by kyphectomy and segmental spinal instrumentation. Heydemann JS, Gillespie R. *Spine* 1987;12:37-41.

> Short-term review of 12 patients treated by kyphectomy and segmental spinal instrumentation. The authors present a method of anterior fixation of the pelvis.

The long-term results of kyphectomy and spinal stabilization in children with myelomeningocele. McMaster MJ. *Spine* 1988;13:417-424.

> Presents a series of 10 patients treated by kyphectomy and various forms of instrumentation for myelomeningocele kyphosis and followed for a mean of seven years. A long fusion from the mid-thoracic region to the sacrum was necessary to provide long-term stability and to prevent the development of thoracic lordosis. Discusses operative techniques, risks, and complications.

Spinal Muscular Atrophy

Spinal muscular atrophy: Natural history and orthopaedic treatment of scoliosis. Granata C, Merlini L, Magni E, et al. *Spine* 1989;14:760-770.

> The authors report on the natural history of scoliosis in 32 cases of mild spinal muscular atrophy and 31 cases of intermediate spinal muscular atrophy. Spinal deformity usually occurs by age 6 and, if not treated, progression is certain. Bracing may slow curve progression. Early surgical stabilization is recommended to prevent pulmonary compromise and functional loss.

Surgical and functional results of spine fusion in spinal muscular atrophy. Brown JC, Zeller JL, Swank SM, et al. *Spine* 1989;14:763-770.

> Two groups of surgically treated patients are reported. Group I, posterior spinal fusion with Harrington rod instrumentation, had a 35% complication rate at average 9-year follow-up. Group II, posterior spinal fusion with Luque rod instrumentation, had a 16% complication rate at average 3.5-year follow-up. Sitting tolerance was maintained after surgery, but preoperative skill levels were never approached.

Spine fusion in patients with spinal muscular atrophy. Aprin H, Bowen JR, MacEwen GD, et al. *J Bone Joint Surg* 1982;64A:1179-1187.

> Presents results in 22 cases. Discusses surgical indications and results, bracing results, and high failure rates. Fusion may slow deterioration of pulmonary function.

Functional classification and orthopaedic management of spinal muscular atrophy. Evans GA, Drennan JC, Russman BS. *J Bone Joint Surg* 1981;63B:516-522.
> Fifty-four patients are reported based on the severity of neurologic deficit. The more severe the weakness, the earlier is the onset of scoliosis. Spine fusion is the treatment of choice for curves of 60 degrees or more.

Muscular Dystrophy

Progression of scoliosis in Duchenne muscular dystrophy. Smith AD, Koreska J, Moseley CF. *J Bone Joint Surg* 1989;71A:1066-1074.
> Longitudinal study of 51 boys with Duchenne muscular dystrophy followed until death without surgical treatment. All patients developed scoliosis, and severe curves led to difficulty sitting, skin breakdown, and pain. When the curve exceeded 35 degrees, the vital capacity usually was less than 40% of predicted. Spinal arthrodesis should be considered when walking becomes impossible.

Pulmonary function and scoliosis in Duchenne dystrophy. Miller F, Moseley CF, Koreska J, et al. *J Pediatr Orthop* 1988;8:133-137.
> Pulmonary function (% forced vital capacity) declines most rapidly during adolescent growth spurt. Surgery does not influence the rate of pulmonary function deterioration.

The natural history of spine curvature progression in the nonambulatory Duchenne muscular dystrophy patient. Hsu JD. *Spine* 1983;8:771-775.
> When the curve progresses beyond 40 degrees, patients experience loss of sitting balance, decreased sitting tolerance, pain, decreased vital capacity, and need to use hands and arms to prop the body. Surgery is indicated to prevent these problems.

Correlation of scoliosis and pulmonary function in Duchenne muscular dystrophy. Kurz, LT, Mubarak SJ, Schultz P, et al. *J Pediatr Orthop* 1983;3:347-353.
> Forced vital capacity peaks at the age when standing ceases. Pulmonary function decreases by 4% each year and with each 10-degree increase in curvature. Early spinal instrumentation is indicated in order to slow deterioration of pulmonary function.

Post Laminectomy Spinal Deformity

Post laminectomy kyphosis and scoliosis in children with spinal tumors. Dietrich U, Schirmer M, Veltrup K, et al. *Neuro Orthop* 1989;7:36-42.
> Nineteen of 22 patients treated by laminectomy in infancy and childhood for spinal tumors developed spinal deformity. Kyphosis developed in 14 cases and scoliosis in 15 cases. The incidence of kyphosis was

highest when the site of laminectomy was in the cervical spine and lowest when it was in the lumbar spine. Resection of facet joints increased the risk of spinal deformity. Careful follow-up and early treatment is indicated for these patients.

The incidence of spinal-column deformity after multiple-level laminectomy in children and adults. Yasuoka S, Peterson HA, MacCarty CS. *J Neurosurg* 1982;57:441-445.
> Discusses the problem of post-laminectomy spinal deformity in a review of 58 patients.

Post-laminectomy kyphosis. Lonstein JE. *Clin Orthop* 1977;128:93-100.
> This excellent review article covers all aspects of post-laminectomy kyphotic deformity and emphasizes the importance of facet-joint integrity.

Neurofibromatosis

Scoliosis in neurofibromatosis: The natural history with and without operation. Calvert PT, Edgar MA, Webb PJ. *J Bone Joint Surg* 1989;71B:246-251.
> Review of 47 patients with neurofibromatosis and dystrophic spinal deformities. Short angular thoracic curves are the commonest pattern. Deterioration is usual, but the rate is unpredictable. Early surgical stabilization by combined anterior and posterior fusion is indicated for kyphotic deformities or dystrophic apical vertebral changes. Selected cases may require posterior fusion and instrumentation alone.

Pitfalls of spinal deformities associated with neurofibromatosis in children. Crawford AH. *Clin Orthop* 1989;245:29-42.
> Excellent review article on all aspects of spinal deformity in neurofibromatosis based on a series of 116 patients. Excellent bibliography.

Neurofibromatosis hyperkyphosis: A review of 33 patients with kyphosis of 80 degrees or greater. Winter RB, Lonstein JE, Anderson M. *J Spinal Disorders* 1988;1:39-49.
> Reviews the natural history of the untreated deformity and the results of treatment. Outlines a plan of management for these patients.

Spine deformity in neurofibromatosis: A review of one hundred and two patients. Winter RB, Moe JH, Bradford DS, et al. *J Bone Joint Surg* 1979;61A:677-694.
> Discussion of problems of spinal deformity (scoliosis and kyphosis) in patients with neurofibromatosis.

Skeletal Dysplasia

Spinal disorders of dwarfism: Review of the literature and report of eighty cases. Bethem D, Winter RB, Lutter L, et al. *J Bone Joint Surg* 1981;63A:1412-1425.
> Review of spinal deformities in patients with osteochondrodystrophies. Discusses diagnosis and management.

Spinal deformity in short-stature syndromes. Tolo VT. In Greene WB (ed): American Academy of Orthopaedic Surgeons *Instructional Course Lectures, XXXIX* . Park Ridge, IL, American Academy of Orthopaedic Surgeons, 1990, pp 399-405.
> This chapter outlines the spine deformities and their treatment in several skeletal dysplasias (achondroplasia, diastrophic dysplasia, pseudoachondroplasia, spondyloepiphyseal dysplasia congenita and tarda, and mucopolysaccharidosis). This chapter is well-referenced and also has the perspective of the author's considerable experience with these uncommon problems.

Herniated Nucleus Pulposa

Lumbar disc excision in children and adolescents. DeOrio JK, Bianco AJ Jr. *J Bone Joint Surg* 1982;64A:991-996.
> Report on diskectomy in children under age 16. Discusses problems of disk herniation in children.

Friedreich's Ataxia

Natural history of scoliosis in Friedreich's ataxia. Labelle H, Tohmé S, Duhaime M, et al. *J Bone Joint Surg* 1986;68A:564-572.
> A study of 56 patients with Friedreich's ataxia revealed that all developed scoliosis and two thirds developed hyperkyphosis. There was no correlation between significant curve progression and duration of disease, ambulatory function, or degree of muscle weakness. Scoliosis in Friedreich's ataxia behaves like idiopathic scoliosis. Includes guidelines for treatment.

Incidence, natural history, and treatment of scoliosis in Friedreich's ataxia. Cady RB, Bobechko WP. *J Pediatr Orthop* 1984;4:673-676.
> Study of 42 patients with Friedreich's ataxia. The incidence of scoliosis is high. Curves tend to progress with disease severity. Bracing has no role in treatment. Early surgical stabilization is indicated in progressive curves.

Arthrogryposis

Spinal deformities in patients with arthrogryposis: A review of 16 patients.
Daher YH, Lonstein JE, Winter RB, et al. *Spine* 1985;10:609-613.
> Literature review and results of management of a small group of patients
> with arthrogryposis.

Prader-Willi Syndrome

Scoliosis surgery in the Prader-Willi Syndrome. Rees D, Jones MW, Owen R,
et al. *J Bone Joint Surg* 1989;71B:685-688.
> Discussion of problems encountered in scoliosis surgery in children with
> Prader-Willi syndrome.

Scoliosis in the Prader-Willi syndrome. Soriano RM, Weisz I, Houghton GR.
Spine 1988;13:209-211.
> Scoliosis occurs in 62% to 86% of patients with Prader-Willi syndrome.
> Authors report on management of five cases.

Spondylolysis and Spondylolisthesis

Current concepts review: Spondylolysis and spondylolisthesis in children and
adolescents. Hensinger RN. *J Bone Joint Surg* 1989;71A:1098-1107.
> Excellent review article covering all aspects of the topic. Includes an
> extensive bibliography.

Non-operative treatment for painful adolescent spondylolysis or
spondylolisthesis. Pizzutillo PD, Hummer CD. *J Pediatr Orthop* 1989;9:538-
540.
> Authors demonstrate symptomatic relief of pain in two thirds of patients
> with spondylolysis and grade I and II spondylolisthesis treated without
> surgery. Adolescents with symptomatic grade III and grade IV
> spondylolisthesis are more appropriately treated surgically.

Spinal arthrodesis for severe spondylolisthesis in children and adolescents: A
long-term follow-up study. Freeman BL III, Donati NL. *J Bone Joint Surg*
1989;71A:594-598.
> Twelve-year follow-up of 12 patients with grade III or grade IV
> spondylolisthesis. Demonstrates that posterior in situ arthrodesis is
> effective, reliable, and safe for treatment of severe spondylolisthesis.

Spondylolisthesis in children under 12 years of age: Long-term results of 56
patients treated conservatively or operatively. Seitsalo S, Osterman K, Poussa
M, et al. *J Pediatr Orthop* 1988;8:516-521.
> Review of 32 surgical and 24 nonsurgical cases of spondylolisthesis.
> Risk factors include female sex and dysplastic olisthesis. Lumbosacral

fusions in situ give good long-term results (average follow-up 14.5 years), despite 16% nonunions and 19% postoperative slip progression.

Closed reduction of spondylolisthesis. An experience in 22 patients. Bradford DS. *Spine* 1988;13:580-587.
> Review of 22 patients with spondylolisthesis treated by closed reduction and posterolateral arthrodesis and followed an average of 40 months. Discusses methods, results, complications, and indications.

Long-term clinical and radiological follow-up of spondylolysis and spondylolisthesis. Saraste H. *J Pediatr Orthop* 1987;7:631-638.
> Long term (mean 29 years) clinical and radiographic follow-up of 255 patients with spondylolisthesis and spondylolysis (13% were less than 15 years of age at diagnosis). Of these patients, 70% had been treated for low back symptoms.

Long-term follow-up of patients with grade-III and IV spondylolisthesis: Treatment with and without posterior fusion. Harris IE, Weinstein SL. *J Bone Joint Surg* 1987;69A:960-969.
> An eighteen-year follow-up of 11 patients with grade III and grade IV spondylolisthesis treated without surgery is compared with a 24-year follow-up of 21 surgically treated patients. The surgical group were less symptomatic and less restricted in their activity than the nonsurgical group. In situ fusion gave good functional long-term results in grade III and grade IV spondylolisthesis.

Lytic spondylolysis: Repair by wiring. Nicol RO, Scott JH. *Spine* 1986;11:1027-1030.
> Describes and gives early results for a technique of defect repair without facet joint sacrifice.

The natural history of spondylolysis and spondylolisthesis. Fredrickson BE, Baker D, McHolick WJ, et al. *J Bone Joint Surg* 1984;66A:699-707.
> Prospective study of 500 unselected first grade children (1955 - 1957) and their families, discussing incidence, relationship of listhesis to lysis, and etiology.

Management of severe spondylolisthesis in children and adolescents. Boxall D, Bradford DS, Winter RB, et al. *J Bone Joint Surg* 1979;61A:479-495.
> Reviews 43 patients with a slip of 50% or more. Discusses the importance of slip angle in addition to percent of slip, and presents the results of fusion.

Reduction of severe spondylolisthesis: A preliminary report. McPhee IB, O'Brien JP. *Spine* 1979;4:430-434.
> Presents a technique of staged reduction.

Surgical management of spondylolisthesis in children and adolescents. Hensinger RN, Lang JR, MacEwen GD. *Spine* 1976;1:207-216.

Four year follow-up on 20 patients undergoing bilateral posterolateral fusion for symptomatic spondylolisthesis. Results are presented and compared with other reported series.

Spondylolysis and spondylolisthesis in children and teen-agers. Turner RH, Bianco AJ Jr. *J Bone Joint Surg* 1971;53A:1298-1306.
Review of eight-year experience in 173 patients. Results of surgical and nonsurgical management are presented. Indications for both kinds of treatment are discussed.

Spondylolisthesis in children. Wiltse LL. *Clin Orthop* 1961;21:156-163.
Discussion of etiology, treatment options, and techniques in spondylolisthesis in children.

Upper-Extremity Deformities

Richard E. McCarthy, MD

Congenital Pseudarthrosis of the Clavicle

Severe complication of surgical treatment of congenital pseudarthrosis of the clavicle. Toledo LC, MacEwen GD. *Clin Orthop* 1979;139:64-67.
>   Neuropraxia of brachial plexus is reported as a complication of surgical treatment.

Congenital pseudarthrosis of the clavicle. Gibson DA, Carroll N. *J Bone Joint Surg* 1970;52B:629-643.
>   Presents clinical findings on 13 patients and discusses etiology and treatment.

Congenital pseudarthrosis of the clavicle. Owen R. *J Bone Joint Surg* 1970;52B:644-652.
>   Reviews 33 cases and discusses methods of treatment.

Congenital pseudarthrosis of the clavicle: A review of the literature and surgical results of six cases. Schnall SB, King JD, Marrero G. *J Pediatr Orthop* 1988;8:316-321.
>   Six patients treated by bone grafting and plate fixation had good results.

Cleidocranial Dysostosis

Cleidocranial dysostosis: The hereditary aspects. Outland T, Sherk HH. *Clin Orthop* 1961;20:241-244.
>   Describes a family in which spontaneous appearance of cleidocranial dysostosis was transmitted to the next generation.

Cranio-cleido-dysostosis. Fairbank HAT. *J Bone Joint Surg* 1949;31B:608-617.
>   Reviews the author's 11 cases and the literature. The clinical presentation is discussed but not the treatment. Associated findings include deficient ossification of the pubis, coxa vara, spina bifida occulta, and long second metacarpal.

Radio-ulnar and Radio-humeral Synostosis

Congenital radioulnar synostosis. Simmons BP, Southmayd WW, Riseborough EJ. *J Hand Surg* 1983;8:829-838.
>   Reviews 33 patients, of whom 20 underwent surgery. Good results were reported in 82%. Osteotomy through the synostosis was the easiest and most reliable procedure. Any derotation greater than 85 degrees should be done in two stages and special attention must be given to vascular status.

Congenital radio-ulnar synostosis: Surgical treatment. Green WT, Mital MA. *J Bone Joint Surg* 1979;61A:738-743.
>   Results of operative approach in 13 patients treated with transverse osteotomy through conjoined radius and ulna. Ideal positions for unilateral and bilateral involvement discussed.

Congenital proximal radio-ulnar synostosis: Clinical and anatomical features. Dal Monte A, Andrisano A, Bungaro P, et al. *Ital J Orthop Traumatol* 1987;13:201-206.
>   The authors analyzed 26 patients having three types of synostoses, most commonly affecting the left side. The type 1 synostosis (partial) had an ossific nucleus present in the radial head without bowing of the forearm. Type 2 synostosis (complete), the most common type, demonstrated forward bowing of the radius, distal subluxation, and absence of the radial head ossific nucleus. Type 3 synostosis (extended) was uncommon and involved the interosseous membrane throughout most of forearm.

A critical review of the surgical treatment of congenital proximal radio-ulnar synostosis. Dal Monte A, Andrisano A, Mignani G, et al. *Ital J Orthop Traumatol* 1987;13:181-186.
>   Treatment results in 26 patients were reviewed. Pronation under 30 degrees (type 1) should not be corrected. Pronation of 30 to 60 degrees should be corrected in the setting of bilaterality, poor cosmetic appearance, involvement of dominant side, or lack of compensatory mechanisms. The ideal age is between 4 and 5 years of age. Resection doesn't work; osteotomies proximally or distally work equally as well and double osteotomies are good for more severe cases. Unilateral cases should be placed beteen 10 and 20 degrees of supination. Bilateral cases should be placed with the dominant forearm in slight pronation and the opposite in slight supination.

Congenital radio-ulnar synostosis: Compensatory rotation around the wrist and rotation osteotomy. Ogino T, Hikino K. *J Hand Surg* 1987;12B:173-178.
>   Patients with pronated forearms with a mean pronation of 60 degrees complained of disability. All patients had compensatory wrist hyperlaxity. Rotational osteotomies done through the fusion mass had good results.

Congenital Dislocation of the Radial Head

Congenital dislocation of the radial head: Spectrum and natural history. Kelly DW. *J Pediatr Orthop* 1981;1:295-298.
> A retrospective review of 24 patients with natural history, associated problems, and results of treatment. Increased ulnar length in relation to radius was a significant diagnostic sign. Radial head excision after age 15 relieved pain and improved cosmesis, but did not yield increased motion.

Developmental posterior dislocation of the radial head. Good CJ, Wicks MH. *J Bone Joint Surg* 1983;65B:64-65.
Unilateral posterior dislocation of the radial head in identical twins. Gattey PH, Wedge JH. *J Pediatr Orthop* 1986;6:220-221.
> These two articles question some of the thinking on congenital dislocations versus developmental dislocations. The authors question whether some unilateral dislocations could be congenital rather than traumatic and whether congenital deformities of the radial head predispose to later subluxations.

Madelung's Deformity

Clinical variation in dyschondrosteosis: A report on 13 individuals in 8 families. Dawe C, Wynne-Davies R, Fulford GE. *J Bone Joint Surg* 1982;64B:377-381.
> Madelung's deformity was the most frequent feature in dyschondrosteosis, and no patient required treatment.

Madelung's deformity: A clinical and cytogenetic study. Henry A, Thorburn MJ. *J Bone Joint Surg* 1967;49B:66-73.
> The deformity is classified into four groups based on etiology. Most patients did not require surgery.

Radial Clubhand (Radial Aplasia)

Centralization of the radial club hand: An ulnar surgical approach. Manske PR, McCarroll HR Jr, Swanson K. *J Hand Surg* 1981;6:423-433.
> The transverse ulnar approach in 22 hands gave stable carpoulnar pseudoarthrosis in 20.

Treatment of congenital deformities of the hand and forearm (first of two parts). Smith RJ, Lipke RW. *N Engl J Med* 1979;300:344-349.
> Surgical treatment of radial clubhand is discussed as is thumb aplasia and vascularized autogenous grafts.

Radial club hand: A continuing study of sixty-eight patients with one hundred and seventeen club hands. Lamb DW. *J Bone Joint Surg* 1977;59A:1-13.

Etiology is discussed. Centralization of the carpus on the ulna gave satisfactory improvement.

Anomalies associated with radial dysplasia. Carroll RE, Louis DS. *J Pediatr* 1974;84:409-411.

A retrospective study of other anomalies associated with radial dysplasia in a series of 53 patients. The majority of these were apparent at birth or shortly thereafter.

Orthopaedic aspects of the VATER association. Lawhon SM, MacEwen GD, Bunnell WP. *J Bone Joint Surg* 1986;68A:424-429.

There are many orthopaedic problems associated with VATER (vertebral, anal, tracheoesophageal, renal, and radial limb anomalies) syndrome. The upper-extremity syndrome deformities include radial aplasia which can involve a spectrum from mild thumb deformities to a complete radial hemimelia. The authors recommend prompt treatment of the orthopaedic problems because the overall prognosis for physical and intellectual development is good.

Radialization as a new treatment for radial club hand. Buck-Gramcko D. *J Hand Surg* 1985;10A:964-968.

The author, a noted authority in radial hemimelia, repositions the hand on the forearm without resection of carpal bones. Surgical correction is maintained by temporarily fixing the hand in ulnar deviation by a Kirschner wire.

Long-term review of the surgical treatment of radial deficiencies. Bayne LG, Klug MS. *J Hand Surg* 1987;12A:169-179.

The author reviews surgical results of a large experience (64 patients, 101 radial deficiencies). The best results occurred with adequate preoperative stretching, central positioning of the hand on the ulna, and postoperative bracing. The ideal age for surgery is between 6 months and 1 year.

A centralization procedure for radial clubhand. Watson HK, Beebe RD, Cruz NI. *J Hand Surg* 1984;9A:541-547.

Twelve centralizations were done with release of fibrotic radial anlage through two z-plasty incisions. There was no resection of carpal bones and the authors reported good results at 10-year follow-up.

Ulnar Aplasia

Functional status in ulnar deficiency. Blair WF, Shurr DG, Buckwalter JA. *J Pediatr Orthop* 1983;3:37-40.

The upper-extremity function of eight untreated patients was evaluated and did not correlate well with radiographic appearance or classification.

Deformities of the hand and wrist with ulnar deficiency. Broudy AS, Smith RJ. *J Hand Surg* 1979;4:304-315.

> Reviews 20 patients with associated deformities of hand and elbow and gives results of surgical treatment.

Anomalies of Hand and Fingers

Toe transfers for congenital hand defects. Gilbert A. *J Hand Surg* 1982;7:118-124.

> The technique and results of microvascular transfer of the second toes in 21 cases is reported. Normal growth of the transfer was found.

Annular constricting bands. Moses JM, Flatt AE, Cooper RR. *J Bone Joint Surg* 1979;61A:562-565.

> Reviews 45 patients with associated problems and gives results of surgical treatment.

Treatment of congenital deformities of the hand and forearm (second of two parts). Smith RJ, Lipke RW. *N Engl J Med* 1979;300:402-407.

> Reviews the surgical and nonsurgical management of congenital hand deformities.

Evaluation of the operative treatment of syndactyly. Toledo LC, Ger E. *J Hand Surg* 1979;4:556-564.

> Reviews surgical treatment of 61 patients.

Macrodactyly. Barsky AJ. *J Bone Joint Surg* 1967;49A:1255-1266.

> In this historical review of macrodactyly, the author expresses discouragement with the results of surgical treatment.

Cleft hand: Classification, incidence, and treatment. Review of the literature and report of nineteen cases. Barsky AJ. *J Bone Joint Surg* 1964;46A:1707-1720.

> This historical review offers a classification and methods of treatment for cleft hand.

Terminal limb congenital malformations: Analysis of 523 cases. Masada K, Tsuyuguchi Y, Kawabata H, et al. *J Pediatr Orthop* 1986;6:340-345.

> Large series looking at the interrelation of hands and feet with terminal malformations.

Early surgical intervention in Apert's syndactyly. Barot LR, Caplan HS. *Plast Reconstr Surg* 1986;77:282-287.

> This paper discusses the technique for early separation of the fingers in children with complex deformities associated with Apert's disease. The authors note their frustration with long-term poor function due to limitation of motion and finger function in spite of improved aesthetic appearance.

Severe limb deficiency in Poland's syndrome. Gausewitz SH, Meals RA, Setoguchi Y. *Clin Orthop* 1984;185;9-13.

>Ten patients were analyzed and classified by a system based on the degree of limb deficiency.

Surgical management of arthrogryposis in the upper extremity. Bennett JB, Hansen PE, Granberry WM, et al. *J Pediatr Orthop* 1985;5:281-286.

>Good overall discussion of the topic. The authors emphasize individualization of the treatment and report moderate success with the majority of cases including derotational osteotomies of the humerus, elbow releases and flexor muscle transfers, correction of thumb-in-palm deformity and wrist flexion deformity with transfers and releases.

Arthrogryposis of the hand. Yonenobu K, Tada K, Swanson AB. *J Pediatr Orthop* 1984;4:599-603.

>Forty-five patients were aggressively treated at an early age with 29 undergoing successful surgery to improve function. They recommended early surgery with releases, muscle transfers, and osteotomies.

Hand assessment and management of arthrogryposis multiplex congenita. Bayne LG. *Clin Orthop* 1985;194:68-73.

>Early treatment of children with arthrogrypotic hand deformities consists of passive stretching, sometimes accompanied by plaster casts or splints. Surgical release of contracted parts can be helpful, as can tendon transfers. Surgical correction of the joints of the hand has not proven very successful. This article provides a succinct look at this difficult area.

Congenital constriction band syndrome. Tada K, Yonenobu K, Swanson AB. *J Pediatr Orthop* 1984;4:726-730.

>Eighty-three patients with congenital constriction band syndrome were analyzed. The distal portion of the extremity was typically involved. The central digits were more frequently constricted and the thumb only minimally involved. Constriction bands, amputation, and acrosyndactyly were the main clinical manifestations of this syndrome. The majority of clubfoot deformities associated with this syndrome were proven to be caused by paralytic clubfoot from compression neuropathy.

Anomalies of the Thumb

Duplication of the thumb: A retrospective review of two hundred and thirty-seven cases. Tada K, Yonenobu K, Tsuyuguchi Y, et al. *J Bone Joint Surg* 1983;65A:584-598.

>Reviews 237 cases treated surgically. The authors found muscle balance important. Arthrodesis was used as a salvage operation after skeletal maturity.

Trigger thumbs in children: A review of the natural history and indications for treatment in 105 patients. Dinham JM, Meggitt BF. *J Bone Joint Surg* 1974;56B:153-155.

> A review of natural history and recommended treatment.

Congenital clasped thumb (congenital flexion-adduction deformity of the thumb): A syndrome, not a specific entity. Weckesser EC, Reed JR, Heiple KG. *J Bone Joint Surg* 1968;50A:1417-1428.

> Classifies this disorder into four groups and presents the treatment of each. The authors suggest that this is a syndrome rather than a specific disease entity.

Reconstruction of the hypoplastic thumb. Lister G. *Clin Orthop* 1985;195:52-65.

> This surgeon's guide to the correction of congenital thumb deformities includes a discussion of the Blauth classification for these deformities and good illustrations of the surgical repairs.

Congenital thumb deformities. Wood VE. *Clin Orthop* 1985;195:7-25.

> This excellent review article covers the vast spectrum of unusual types of thumb deformities.

Pediatric Hip

J. Andy Sullivan, MD
Eric Jones, MD

Congenital Dislocation

Congenital Dislocation of the Hip. Tachdjian MO (ed). New York, Churchill Livingstone, 1982.

Congenital dislocation of the hip. Hensinger RN. CIBA *Clin Symp* 1979;31:3-31.

Congenital Dysplasia and Dislocation of the Hip. Coleman SS. St. Louis, CV Mosby, 1978.

Congenital hip dysplasia. Staheli LT, Coleman SS, Hensinger RN, et al. In Murray JA (ed): American Academy of Orthopaedic Surgeons *Instructional Course Lectures, XXXIII*. St. Louis, CV Mosby, 1984, pp 350-363.
> "State of the art" as seen by leading experts of the time.

Diagnosis of congenital dysplasia of the hip in the newborn infant. Coleman SS. *Clin Orthop* 1989;247:3-12. Abridged from: *JAMA* 1956;162:548-554.
> A classic.

Congenital dislocation of the hip: Recent advances and current problems. Bennett JT, MacEwen GD. *Clin Orthop* 1989;247:15-21.
> A good, concise source of information on the diagnosis and management of this condition.

Vascular Supply

The normal vascular anatomy of the human femoral head during growth. Trueta J. *J Bone Joint Surg* 1957;39B:358-394.
> A classic article on blood supply to the developing proximal femur.

The arterial supply of the developing proximal end of the human femur. Chung SM. *J Bone Joint Surg* 1976;58A:961-970.
> Perfusion studies done in 150 autopsy specimens of children age 26 weeks of gestation to age 14 years. Two anastomotic rings were formed by the medial and lateral circumflex femoral arteries. Vessels ascended to enter the capital epiphysis via the perichondral ring. The major blood

supply to the head and neck of the femur came from lateral ascending cervical branches of the extracapsular ring, predominantly supplied by the medial circumflex femoral artery. Variations of distribution were found with age, sex, and race. The epiphyseal plate was an absolute barrier to blood vessels in all but two cases. The arteries of the ligamentum teres were inconsistently present.

Changing patterns of proximal femoral vascularity. Ogden JA. *J Bone Joint Surg* 1974; 56A:941-950.

Thirty-six autopsy specimens of children age 7 months of gestation to age 3 years were studied. Initially the proximal femoral chondroepiphysis and growth plate are supplied approximately equally by the lateral circumflex system and the medial circumflex system. Later the lateral system regresses and the medial circumflex system becomes the predominant source. Differential growth of the proximal femur was a significant factor in changing this distribution.

Early Diagnosis and Treatment

Efficacy of neonatal hip examination. Tredwell SJ, Bell HM. *J Pediatr Orthop* 1981;1:61-65.

Of live births, 9.8 per 1000 have unstable hips. Treatment was immediate splinting in flexion and abduction for a few days to two months. A few cases required adductor release and spica cast. None needed open reduction. There was one false negative screening, and five who later presented with adduction contracture and acetabular dysplasia despite a normal neonatal examination.

Neonatal screening for congenital dislocation of the hip: A prospective 21-year survey. Hadlow V. *J Bone Joint Surg* 1988;70B:740-743.

Reports a prospective study of 20,657 babies with an incidence of instability of 672 (3.2%). Two cases were undetected until the ages 15 months and 18 months.

Clinical assessment of hip instability in the newborn by an orthopedic surgeon and a pediatrician. Bialik V, Fishman J, Katzir J, et al. *J Pediatr Orthop* 1986;6:703-705.

This is a very important article with regard to understanding and evaluating hip screening. One cannot detect all cases of congenital hip dysplasia at birth. In this study a pediatric orthopaedist, a neonatal pediatrician, and a pediatrician, each working independently, examined the babies. Each independent examiner was able to detect 51 babies that had neonatal hip instability; however, in an additional 25 babies, one of the examiners failed to detect this instability at initial examination. In addition, 36 babies whose hips were stable at birth later required orthopaedic treatment for congenital hip dysplasia. Screening for neonatal hip dysplasia must be dynamic and progressive and should continue throughout the first year of life or until walking age.

Problems in early recognition of hip dysplasia. Davies SJ, Walker G. *J Bone Joint Surg* 1984;66B:479-484.

> Ten children who had stable hips at birth were later found to have acetabular dysplasia. Four went on to late dislocation. The conclusion is that some cases of hip dysplasia have an etiology different from that of hips that are unstable at birth. Cases of late detected hip dislocations were not necessarily missed at neonatal examination.

Missed or developmental dislocation of the hip. Ilfeld W, Westin GW, Makin M. *Clin Orthop* 1986;203:276-281.

> This important article documents that patients diagnosed with subluxation or dislocation of the hip were discovered months or years after previous multiple examinations by physicians specializing in children's orthopaedics. Delayed diagnosis of dislocation is not evidence that an inadequate physical examination was performed. Examinations need to be performed repeatedly throughout the first two years of life.

Early diagnosis and treatment of congenital dislocation of the hip. Barlow TG. *J Bone Joint Surg* 1962;44B:292-301.

> Describes a test for instability of the hip in the newborn that is more sensitive than Ortolani's. Of unstable hips, 88% recover in the first week or first 2 months of life. The remainder persist unless treated.

Imaging

Arthrography in the evaluation of congenital dislocation of the hip. Drummond DS, O'Donnell J, Breed A, et al. *Clin Orthop* 1989;243:148-156.

> Reviews 48 preoperative hip arthrograms of 35 children under 18 months of age who were treated for congenital dysplasia of the hip. Other imaging modalities are reviewed, and the authors conclude that arthrography is the benchmark study for congenital dislocation of the hip.

Ultrasound screening of hips at risk for CDH: Failure to reduce the incidence of late cases. Clarke NMP, Clegg J, Al-Chalabi AN. *J Bone Joint Surg* 1989:71B:9-12.

> Ultrasound examination can be an accurate method of diagnosing congenital dislocation of the hip in infancy. It is neither cost effective nor practical to screen all infants. In this study, the authors screened only infants considered to be at risk as well as those with hip abnormalities detected on clinical exam. Seventeen (3.7 per thousand) required treatment. In five of these, no clinical abnormality had been detected. Eighty-one patients had ultrasound abnormalities but did not require treatment despite the fact that ultrasound at first showed major hip displacement in seventeen. Three late cases of undiagnosed congenital dislocation of the hip are presented that had not been detected by ultrasound. The authors conclude that, compared with the previous

nine years, the incidence of late congenital dislocation of the hip is unchanged.

Fundamentals of sonographic diagnosis of infant hip dysplasia. Graf R. *J Pediatr Orthop* 1984;4:735-740.
>Sonography (ultrasonography) has been touted as a noninvasive nonradiating means of diagnosing infants with hip dysplasia and dislocation. This article reports examinations of 3,500 infants, describes the technique, outlines the author's classification system, and discusses indications for its use. Sonography is not practical for screening all newborns.

Ultrasonography in developmental displacement of the hip: A critical analysis of our results. Bialik V, Reuveni A, Pery M, et al. *J Pediatr Orthop* 1989;9:154-156.
>Ultrasonographic examinations (1,008) were performed on 444 hips. Sixty-nine randomly selected infants, 25 babies at risk, and 125 infants with hip pathology were examined. Specificity, selectivity, and predictive values of real-time sector scanning were evaluated. Real-time sector scanning was not proven to be an absolute imaging method.

The use of computerised tomography in dislocation of the hip and femoral neck anteversion in children. Peterson HA, Klassen RA, McLeod RA, et al. *J Bone Joint Surg* 1981;63B:198-208.
>This technique needs to be used selectively because of the expense and the high gonadal radiation doses. Criteria for use are problems in the hips of children older than 18 months of age whose range of movement is limited or who have osseous changes that make examination and assessment by standard radiographic techniques incomplete.

Three-dimensional digital display in congenital dislocations of the hips: Preliminary experience. Lange P, Genant HK, Steiger P, et al. *J Pediatr Orthop* 1989;9:532-537.
>Reports four patients with congenital dislocation of the hip studied with three-dimensional computerized tomography or three-dimensional magnetic resonance imaging. These techniques appear promising in confirming a diagnosis and in facilitating the choice of treatment. The results are preliminary.

Magnetic resonance imaging in congenital dislocation of the hip. Bos CF, Bloem JL, Obermann WR, et al. *J Bone Joint Surg* 1988;70B:174-178.
>Reviews results of magnetic resonance imaging studies of 15 hips in ten patients with congenital dislocation. Anatomic result is shown as well as the anatomic structures. Two patients required general anesthesia; the others were sedated. Indications, advantages, and disadvantages are given.

Closed Treatment

Prospective study of congenital dislocation of the hip. Tredwell SJ, Davis LA. *J Pediatr Orthop* 1989;9:386-390.
> This prospective study looks at 62 newborns diagnosed as having subluxable or dislocatable hips. It emphasizes the need to treat such cases from birth and provides a treatment cascade. The authors achieved a 100% success rate with no iatrogenic complications.

Stirrups as an aid in the treatment of congenital dysplasias of the hip in children. Pavlik A. *J Pediatr Orthop* 1989;9:157-159.
> This translation of Dr. Pavlik's article from 1950 describes his experience in use of the Pavlik harness.

Congenital dislocation of the hip: Use of the Pavlik harness in the child during the first six months of life. Ramsey PL, Lasser S, MacEwen GD. *J Bone Joint Surg* 1976;58A:1000-1004.
> A classic description of the method.

Treatment of congenital dislocation of the hips by the Pavlik harness: Mechanism of reduction and usage. Iwasaki K. *J Bone Joint Surg* 1983;65A:760-767.
> Avascular necrosis of the femoral head developed in 7% of patients treated at home and in 28% of patients treated in hospital (where a rigid positioning technique was followed). To safely use this simple device, one must understand its proper application and avoid forced positions.

The Pavlik harness: Results in patients over three months of age. Kalamchi A, MacFarlane R III. *J Pediatr Orthop* 1982;2:3-8.
> In 122 older patients, there were 25 dislocations and 114 dysplastic hips. Three dislocated hips required open reduction. The remainder had good results, with no cases of avascular necrosis.

Pitfalls in the use of the Pavlik harness for treatment of congenital dysplasia, subluxation, and dislocation of the hip. Mubarak S, Garfin S, Vance R, et al *J Bone Joint Surg* 1981;63A:1239-1248.
> The most common difficulty was failure to achieve reduction or to recognize that it had not been achieved. Specific recommendations are given for strap adjustment and for the overall management plan.

Noncompliance with Pavlik harness treatment of the infantile hip problems. McHale KA, Corbett D. *J Pediatr Orthop* 1989;9:649-652.
> Reviews use and parental compliance with the Pavlik harness in 27 patients. Outlines problems in the use of the harness.

Home traction in the management of congenital dislocation of the hips. Mubarak SJ, Beck LR, Sutherland D. *J Pediatr Orthop* 1986;6:721-723.
> Children requiring treatment for congenital dislocation of the hip are said to benefit from preoperative traction to reduce the complication of

avascular necrosis of the capital femoral epiphysis. Home traction programs have been instituted to reduce the period of hospitalization and thereby the cost. The article describes an inexpensive technique using a lightweight polyvinyl chloride frame.

Treatment of congenital dislocation of the hip in children between the ages of one and three years. Zionts LE, MacEwen GD. *J Bone Joint Surg* 1986;68A:829-846.

Reviews 51 congenitally dislocated hips in 42 children between 1 and 3 years of age. Treatment used traction, gentle closed reduction under anesthesia, selected adductor tenotomy, and immobilization in the hip spica cast. Of the 51, 25% required open reduction when stable closed reduction could not be achieved. Concludes that in this age group congenital dislocation of the hips is best treated by closed reduction followed by femoral or acetabular procedures at a later date if needed. Open reduction is reserved for hips that cannot be reduced by closed means. Results were excellent in 90% of hips. Significant avascular necrosis developed in three hips, only one of which had been treated by closed reduction. The acetabulum continued to remodel for up to six years after reduction.

CDH diagnosed at 2 to 12 months of age: Treatment and results. Strömqvist B, Sundén G. *J Pediatr Orthop* 1989;9:208-212.

Presents a treatment program of skin traction, arthrography, adductor tenotomy, and psoas tenotomy with immobilization in frog position with plaster cast for 8 to 12 weeks, followed by abduction frame.

Triple prevention of congenital dislocation of the hip. Klisic P, Rakic K, Pajic D. *J Pediatr Orthop* 1984;4:759-761.

This article acknowledges that not all dislocations of the hip can be detected at birth. Recommends an approach that includes examination of newborns to detect symptomatic suspected cases as early as possible. Suggests that all asymptomatic newborns and infants be diapered in abduction as a routine prophylactic measure. Stresses that all infants must be examined until walking age. Bibliography covers the problem of failure to detect all patients with hip pathology regardless of the examination method used.

Acetabular Development After Reduction

Acetabular development after reduction in congenital dislocation of the hip. Lindstrom JR, Ponseti IV, Wenger DR. *J Bone Joint Surg* 1979;61A:112-118.

Significant and continuing improvement of the acetabular index was observed between two and eight years after reduction when the femoral head remained concentrically reduced. Failure to maintain proper reduction led to poor results, as did necrosis of the femoral head.

Acetabular development in the infant's dislocated hips. Cherney DL, Westin GW. *Clin Orthop* 1989;242:98-103.
> Congenital dislocated hips (105) in 83 children were followed with center edge angles and acetabular indices for an average of eight years after reduction to gauge the response of acetabulum to reduction. Major acetabular response occurred in the first year after reduction in children whose hips were reduced before the age of three, whereas the maximal response in children whose hips were reduced after age three occurred in the second through the fourth years. The authors relate that the postreduction acetabular index is a good prognosticator of children who will later require acetabular reconstructive procedures.

Congenital dislocation of the hip: Prolonged acetabular deficiency in adolescents (absence of the lateral acetabular epiphysis) after limbectomy in infancy. O'Hara JN. *J Pediatr Orthop* 1989;9:640-648.
> Reviews 31 patients who had a limbectomy as part of the treatment of congenital dislocation of the hip. In these the lateral acetabular iliac epiphysis failed to appear by age 13, adversely effecting acetabular development. Concludes that excision of the limbus is avoidable, undesirable, and unnecessary.

Open Reduction

A comparative evaluation of the current methods for open reduction of the congenitally displaced hip. Simons GW. *Orthop Clin North Am* 1980;11:161-181.
> An exhaustive review of the five basic forms of open reduction. The author believes that each of the procedures is well suited for a particular type of case and gives criteria for matching patients with procedures.

Primary open reduction of congenital dislocation of the hip using a median adductor approach. Ferguson AB Jr. *J Bone Joint Surg* 1973;55A:671-689.
> This modification of the Ludloff medial approach to the hip is advocated as a primary procedure (without preoperative traction) in infants under the age of 24 months whose ligaments are sufficiently tight to preclude easy closed reduction.

Congenital dislocation of the hip: Open reduction by the medial approach. Kalamchi A, Schmidt TL, MacEwen GD. *Clin Orthop* 1982;169:127-132.
> This review of cases treated at the AI duPont Institute using the Ferguson variant of medial open reduction found a significantly high rate of avascular necrosis and poor stability of reduction. The authors no longer use this technique in young patients with congenital hip dislocation.

Congenital dislocation of the hip: Open reduction through a medial approach. Weinstein SL, Ponseti IV. *J Bone Joint Surg* 1979;61A:119-124.

The authors approach the hip by going between the pectineus and psoas. The iliopsoas tendon is routinely sectioned. Their experience in 22 hips was generally good with two cases of avascular necrosis and two cases of subsequent instability of reduction.

Pelvic and Femoral Osteotomy

Preoperative roentgenographic evaluation for osteotomies about the hip in children. Rab GT. *J Bone Joint Surg* 1981;63A:306-309.
> Describes a roentgenographic technique that helps predict the value of innominate osteotomy and femoral osteotomy in cases of congenital dislocation of the hip and Legg-Perthes disease.

Innominate osteotomy in the treatment of congenital dislocation and subluxation of the hip. Salter RB. *J Bone Joint Surg* 1961;43B:518-539.
Pericapsular osteotomy of the ilium for treatment of congenital subluxation and dislocation of the hip. Pemberton PA. *J Bone Joint Surg* 1965;47A:65-86.
The first fifteen years' personal experience with innominate osteotomy in the treatment of congenital dislocation and subluxation of the hip. Salter RB, Dubos J-P. *Clin Orthop* 1974;98:72-103.
> Three classic articles.

Innominate osteotomy in the management of residual congenital subluxation of the hip in young adults. Salter RB, Hansson G, Thompson GH. *Clin Orthop* 1984;182:53-68.
> Indications for the Salter innominate osteotomy are extended into the older age group. Describes aims, surgical technique, and results in 53 patients with 57 subluxed hips.

Double innominate osteotomy. Sutherland DH, Greenfield R. *J Bone Joint Surg* 1977;59A:1082-1091.
> Pubic osteotomy is used in older children as an addition to the Salter innominate osteotomy to provide better coverage and medial displacement of the femoral head.

Triple osteotomy of the innominate bone. Steele HH. *J Bone Joint Surg* 1973;55A:343-350.
> Recommended for patients who were not considered candidates for other displacement osteotomies (Salter, Pemberton, or Chiari) or for the arthroplasty of Colonna.

Triple osteotomy of the innominate bone for the treatment of congenital hip dysplasia. Kumar SJ, MacEwen GD, Jaykumar AS. *J Pediatr Orthop* 1986;6:393-398.
> Triple osteotomy of the innominate bone described by Steele is indicated for the adolescent or young adult to redirect the acetabulum in the presence of significant symptomatic acetabular dysplasia. In this series of 11 patients, a shelf was also added, which helped increase the

acetabular angle by an average of 10 degrees. The patient should have an adequate joint space and good range of motion preoperatively.

Medial displacement osteotomy of the pelvis. Chiari K. *Clin Orthop* 1974;98:55-71.
    Classic.

Varus derotation osteotomy in the treatment of persistent dysplasia in congenital dislocation of the hip. Kasser JR, Bowen JR, MacEwen GD. *J Bone Joint Surg* 1985;67A:195-202.
    Defines the indications and limitations of varus derotational osteotomy in the treatment of persistent dysplasia in congenital hip dislocation. Concludes that good results can be obtained in patients younger than 4 years of age with acetabular remodeling continuing to the age of 8. Between 4 and 8 the results are less predictable. Over 8 there is no benefit. Preexisting avascular necrosis compromises the results. Articulation of the femoral head with a false acetabulum is a contraindication to isolated varus osteotomy.

Congenital dislocation of the hip in children: Comparison of the effects of femoral shortening and of skeletal traction in treatment. Schoenecker PL, Strecker WB. *J Bone Joint Surg* 1984;66A:21-27.
    Femoral diaphyseal shortening was found to be preferable to traction as an aid in the surgical reduction of a congenitally dislocated hip in children older than three years of age.

One-stage treatment of congenital dislocation of the hip in older children, including femoral shortening. Galpin RD, Roach JW, Wenger DR, et al. *J Bone Joint Surg* 1989;71A:734-741.
    Reviews the results of primary operative treatment in 25 patients with 33 dislocated hips who were 2 years of age or older at the time of the congenital dislocation of the hip. The procedure consists of open reduction, femoral shortening with rotation and varus when necessary, and pelvic osteotomy when necessary. No preliminary traction was used. Overall, the experience was satisfactory. Three of the hips (10%) developed avascular necrosis that was partial and did not adversely effect the clinical or radiographic result. A satisfactory clinical result was obtained in 85% of the series. Leg-length inequality partially corrected with time and did not pose a major problem.

Complications

Avascular necrosis of the capital femoral epiphysis as a complication of closed reduction of congenital dislocation of the hip: A critical review of twenty years' experiences at Gillette Children's Hospital. Gage JR, Winter RB. *J Bone Joint Surg* 1972;54A:373-388.
    A program of adequate traction, gentle reduction, and avoidance of the extreme Lorenz position reduced the incidence of total avascular necrosis

from 35% to 4.5%. The incidence of partial necrosis remained constant at 15% to 20%.

Inadequate reduction of congenital dislocation of the hip. Renshaw TS. *J Bone Joint Surg* 1981;63A:1114-1121.

Lateral position of the femoral head after reduction can be caused by soft-tissue interposition that does not resolve after prolonged proper positioning. The author advises early arthrography and uses the findings as a basis for deciding if open reduction is needed.

Congenital dislocation of the hip: An evaluation of closed reduction. Race C, Herring JA. *J Pediatr Orthop* 1983;3:166-172.

Poor results can be expected when reduction is not concentric. Parameters for judging reduction are based on plain roentgenograms and arthrograms. Poor reductions cannot be managed by closed means. Mild lateralization of the femoral head at the time of initial reduction can be successfully treated by closed means provided that there is progressive improvement in the acetabular index and coverage of the head by the acetabulum.

Avascular necrosis after open reduction for congenital dislocation of the hip: Analysis of causative factors and natural history. Thomas IH, Dunin AJ, Cole WG, et al. *J Pediatr Orthop* 1989;9:525-531.

Reviews causative factors associated with avascular necrosis after open reduction of 87 dislocated hips. Avascular necrosis was observed in 37%. Only 85% of hips with avascular necrosis had a good late result. The authors believe that open reduction was not a causative factor because it did not affect the incidence of avascular necrosis in hips treated in their institution. Use of traction did not reduce the incidence of avascular necrosis.

Treatment concepts for proximal femoral ischemic necrosis complicating congenital hip disease. Thomas CL, Gage JR, Ogden JA. *J Bone Joint Surg* 1982;64A:817-828.

The Bucholz-Ogden classification is used as the basis for prognosis and treatment.

Avascular necrosis in congenital hip dysplasia: The effect of treatment. Robinson HJ Jr, Shannon MA. *J Pediatr Orthop* 1989;9:293-303.

Reviews 39 patients with 50 involved hips analyzed at a mean age of 25 years. In this series nonoperative maintenance of a reduced femoral head carried the best prognosis. When reduction could not be maintained, early pelvic or femoral osteotomy appeared to have the best prognosis. Also covers late salvage procedures and total joint arthroplasty.

The early identification and classification of growth disturbances of the proximal end of the femur. O'Brien T, Millis MB, Griffin PP. *J Bone Joint Surg* 1986:68A:970-980.

Analyzes serial radiographs of 68 patients treated for congenital dislocation of the hip. If there is going to be a growth disturbance, a line will appear in the proximal femur during the first year of life. The pattern of this line can predict the character of the metaphyseal growth disturbance, which can be classified according to the site and extent of physeal closure. Two typical patterns of premature closure were identified.

Treatment of failed open reduction for congenital dislocation of the hip. McCluskey WP, Basset GS, Mora-Garcia G, et al. *J Pediatr Orthop* 1989;9:633-639.
Reviews 23 patients who had an operation for recurrent or persistent dislocation after a previous attempt at open reduction. The majority of the hips were not concentrically reduced during the first procedure. Common causes of failure were improper closure of the capsule and failure to release the tight inferior capsule and transverse acetabular ligament. Avascular necrosis was documented in 44% of the hips.

Teratologic Dislocation

Teratologic congenital dislocation of the hip: Report of two cases. Aaro S, Gottfries B, Kraepelien T, et al. *Acta Orthop Scand* 1983;54:178-181.
Precise discussion of a little-known subject. Cases from the duPont Institute.

Teratologic dislocation of the hip. Gruel CR, Birch JG, Roach JW, et al. *J Pediatr Orthop* 1986;6:693-702.
Reviews 27 teratologic hip dislocations in 17 patients. Closed reductions fared worse than those treated by surgery. These patients have a high complication rate. Discusses indications for surgery and procedures the authors felt were not successful.

Legg-Calvé-Perthes

Legg-Calvé-Perthes disease: Diagnostic and prognostic techniques. Beaty JH. In Barr JS Jr (ed): American Academy of Orthopaedic Surgeons *Instructional Course Lectures, XXXVIII*. Park Ridge, IL, American Academy of Orthopaedic Surgeons, 1989, pp 291-296.
Legg-Calvé-Perthes disease. Catterall A. In Barr JS Jr (ed): American Academy of Orthopaedic Surgeons *Instructional Course Lectures, XXXVIII*. Park Ridge, IL, American Academy of Orthopaedic Surgeons, 1989, pp 297-303.
Nonsurgical treatment of Legg-Calvé-Perthes disease. Fackler CD. In Barr JS Jr (ed): American Academy of Orthopaedic Surgeons *Instructional Course Lectures Series, XXXVIII*. Park Ridge, IL, American Academy of Orthopaedic Surgeons, 1989, pp 305-308.

Legg-Calvé-Perthes disease: A review of current knowledge. Herring JA. In Barr JS Jr (ed): American Academy of Orthopaedic Surgeons *Instructional Course Lectures, XXXVIII*. Park Ridge, IL, American Academy of Orthopaedic Surgeons, 1989, pp 309-315.

    This series of recent articles, which review the natural history, presentation, diagnostic techniques, and treatment by nonsurgical and surgical means, is a good place to start when learning about Legg-Calvé-Perthes disease.

Legg-Calvé-Perthes disease. Weinstein SL. In Evarts CM (ed): American Acadmy of Orthopaedic Surgeons *Instructional Course Lectures, XXXII*. St. Louis, CV Mosby, 1983, pp 272-291.

    A comprehensive review of the early history, epidemiology, etiology, correlative pathology, prognosis, and results of treatment. Orthotic containment is preferred when treatment is required.

The present status of surgical treatment for Legg-Calvé-Perthes disease. Salter RB. *J Bone Joint Surg* 1984;66A:961-966.

    Treatment concepts are based on the desirability of femoral head containment within the acetabulum combined with weightbearing to prevent deformity. Late surgical treatment to correct existing deformity is also reviewed. Orthotic methods of containment are not discussed. Approximately one half of cases require treatment.

Legg-Calvé-Perthes disease. Histochemical and ultrastructural observations of the epiphyseal cartilage and physis. Ponseti IV, Maynard JA, Weinstein SL, et al. *J Bone Joint Surg* 1983;65A:797-807.

    Suggests the disease could be a localized expression of a generalized transient disorder of the epiphyseal cartilage. The persistence of abnormally soft cartilage through which the blood vessels have to penetrate into the femoral head could cause repeated episodes of ischemia and prolong the disease. It is uncertain whether cartilage abnormalities are primary or secondary to ischemia.

The natural history of Perthes' disease. Catterall A. *J Bone Joint Surg* 1971;53B:37-53.

    A classic description of epiphyseal involvement determined by radiologic appearances. Treatment and prognosis are based on the classification.

Legg-Calvé-Perthes disease: The prognostic significance of the subchondral fracture and a two-group classification of the femoral head involvement. Salter RB, Thompson GH. *J Bone Joint Surg* 1984;66A:479-489.

    Describes the prognostic value of the subchondral fracture as seen on radiographs. Introduces a new classification based on the extent of femoral head involvement: Group A, less than half the head; Group B, more than half the head.

Bone scintigraphy in Perthes disease. Bensahel H, Bok B, Cavailloles F, et al. *J Pediatr Orthop* 1983;3:302-305.

Bone scans after intravenous injection of technetium methyldiphosphonate were abnormal in 86% of children with Perthes disease. There were no false positives. Bone scan was more sensitive than plain radiographs in the early stages of the disease.

Gage's sign--revisited! Schlesinger I, Crider RJ. *J Pediatr Orthop* 1988;8:201-202.

Describes the use of the eponym Gage's sign and attempts to clarify Catterall's description of this radiographic finding, which differs from Gage's original description.

A long-term follow-up of Legg-Calvé-Perthes disease. McAndrew MP, Weinstein SL. *J Bone Joint Surg* 1984;66A:860-869.

Reviews a group of patients treated between 1920 and 1940. Statistically significant correlations were found between clinical outcome and Caterall head-at-risk signs, femoral head-size ratio, and age at onset of the disease. Half of the patients in this study had disabling osteoarthrosis by the time they had reached the sixth decade of life.

Legg-Perthes disease in children less than four years old. Clark TE, Finnegan TL, Fisher RL, et al. *J Bone Joint Surg* 1978;60A:166-168.

Children in this age group have a better prognosis than do older children. Results are better in cases with Catterall III and IV disease if they are treated actively rather than observed without treatment.

Premature epiphysial closure in Perthes' disease. Barnes JM. *J Bone Joint Surg* 1980;62B:432-437.

Premature epiphyseal closure is an infrequent complication of Perthes disease. The most common associated procedure in this group of 22 patients was a varus osteotomy done late in the course of the disease.

Treatment

A comparative study of ambulation abduction bracing and varus derotation osteotomy in the treatment of severe Legg-Calvé-Perthes disease in children over six years of age. Evans IK, Deluca PA, Gage JR. *J Pediatr Orthop* 1988;8:676-682.

Thirty-six patients with severe Legg-Calvé-Perthes disease were reviewed retrospectively to compare the results of ambulation-abduction bracing with varus derotation osteotomy. There were 17 brace patients and 19 osteotomy patients, and all were aged 6 to 9 years. Treatment results were equal. The varus neckshaft angle and leg-length discrepancy resulting from the osteotomy were not permanent.

Innominate osteotomy in Perthes disease. Robinson HJ JR, Putter H, Sigmond MB, et al. *J Pediatr Orthop* 1988;8:426-435.

A retrospective study of 27 patients who underwent innominate osteotomy for the treatment of severe Perthes disease. Follow-up ranged from 5 to 16 years. Preoperative and postoperative periods of treatment were more prolonged than those reported by Salter. Clinically good or fair results were obtained in 88%.

Comparison of femoral and innominate osteotomies for the treatment of Legg-Calvé-Perthes disease. Sponseller PD, Desai SS, Millis MB. *J Bone Joint Surg* 1988;70A:1131-1139.

For patients less than ten years old at the onset of disease, there was no difference in the results of the two procedures. The patients older than 10 years of age at the onset of the disease had a poor result with either procedure.

Slipped Capital Femoral Epiphysis

Principles of in situ fixation in chronic slipped capital femoral epiphysis. Morrissy RT. In Barr JS Jr (ed): American Academy of Orthopaedic Surgeons *Instructional Course Lectures, XXXVIII*. Park Ridge, IL, American Academy of Orthopaedic Surgeons, 1989, pp 257-262.

Bone graft epiphysiodesis in the treatment of slipped capital femoral epiphysis. Weiner DS. In Barr JS Jr (ed): American Academy of Orthopaedic Surgeons *Instructional Course Lectures, XXXVIII*. Park Ridge, IL, American Academy of Orthopaedic Surgeons, 1989, pp 263-272.

The role of osteotomy in the treatment of slipped capital femoral epiphysis. Crawford AH. In Barr JS Jr (ed): American Academy of Orthopaedic Surgeons *Instructional Course Lectures, XXXVIII*. Park Ridge, IL, American Academy of Orthopaedic Surgeons, 1989, pp 273-280.

Problems and complications of slipped capital femoral epiphysis. Canale ST. In Barr JS Jr (ed): American Academy of Orthopaedic Surgeons *Instructional Course Lectures, XXXVIII*. Park Ridge, IL, American Academy of Orthopaedic Surgeons, 1989, pp 281-290.

This recent series of articles on the different surgical options and complications of treating slipped capital femoral epiphysis illuminate the principles and techniques of different surgical options and treatment modalities and reviews the problems and complications of the disease.

The ultrastructure of the growth plate in slipped capital femoral epiphysis. Mickelson MR, Ponseti IV, Cooper RR, et al. *J Bone Joint Surg* 1977;59A:1076-1081.

Core biopsy specimens of three patients with slipped capital femoral epiphysis revealed that the slipping occurred in the hypertrophic zone of the growth plate. Marked disorganization of the chondrocyte columns was seen in some areas. It was not apparent whether this abnormality was secondary to partial mechanical disruption of the growth plate or to another process that causes weakness in the growth plate, predisposing to slipped capital femoral epiphysis.

Shear strength of the human femoral capital epiphyseal plate. Chung SM, Batterman SC, Brighton CT. *J Bone Joint Surg* 1976;58A:94-103.

A cadaver study on post mortem specimens. The shear strength of the epiphyseal plate varied with age and was greatly dependent on the surrounding perichondrial complex, particularly in younger children. The forces necessary to cause slipping were within the physiological range of the force that would be generated in overweight children, suggesting that purely mechanical factors may play a major role in the etiology of slipped capital femoral epiphysis.

Obesity and decreased femoral anteversion in adolescence. Galbraith RT, Gelberman RH, Hajek PC, et al. *J Orthop Res* 1987;5:523-528.
    Compared with children of normal weight, obese children showed a significantly reduced angle of femoral anteversion. This may account for the association of slipped capital femoral epiphysis, reduced femoral anteversion, and obesity in the adolescent population.

Mechanical factors in slipped capital femoral epiphysis. Pritchett JW, Perdue KD. *J Pediatr Orthop* 1988;8:385-388.
    Three-dimensional force analyses on the hips of 50 normal patients and 50 patients with slipped capital femoral epiphysis showed the slipped epiphysis patients have reduced resistance to shear because of increased body weight and a decreased neck shaft-plate angle. Slipped epiphysis patients have relative retroversion, which generates increase sagittal plane shear stress at the proximal femoral growth plate.

Treatment

Comparative study of pinning in situ and open epiphysiodesis in 105 patients with slipped capital femoral epiphyses. Zahrawi FB, Stephens TL, Spencer GE, et al. *Clin Orthop* 1983;177:160-168.
    Pinning in situ was performed on 61 hips and open epiphysiodesis was performed in 33 hips. In situ pinning had 91.7% good or excellent results, whereas the epiphysiodesis produced 71.6% good or excellent results. Concludes that pinning in situ is the treatment of choice.

Remodeling of the femoral neck after in situ pinning for slipped capital femoral epiphysis. O'Brien ET, Fahey JJ. *J Bone Joint Surg* 1977:59A:62-68.
    Of 62 patients, 12 had moderate or severe slipping. All were treated with in situ pinning. All but two patients had satisfactory remodeling of the femoral head and neck and were asymptomatic. More difficult procedures, such as osteotomy at the level of the lesser trochanter or neck osteoplasty, may be reserved for the few cases where satisfactory remodeling does not occur.

Treatment of chronic slipped capital femoral epiphysis by bone-grafted epiphyseodesis. Melby A, Hoyt WA Jr, Weiner DS. *J Bone Joint Surg* 1980;62A:119-125.

Bone-graft epiphysiodesis produced rapid and reliable growth-plate closure in the slipped capital femoral epiphysis. Iliac bone is packed in cylindrical holes created with a hollow drill. No cast is used.

Treatment of slipped capital femoral epiphysis by epiphyseodesis and osteoplasty of the femoral neck: A report of further experiences. Herndon CH, Heyman CH, Bell DM. *J Bone Joint Surg* 1963:45A:999-1012.

A classic article favoring in situ epiphysiodesis in all cases of slipped capital femoral epiphysis with reshaping of the femoral neck in more severe deformity. Results were superior to those reported after internal fixation and much better than those reported after repositioning of the femoral head. (Editor's note: Osteoplasty is less often performed since the discovery that a considerable amount of spontaneous remodeling occurs.)

Treatment of slipped upper femoral epiphysis: 80 cases operated on over 10 years (1968-1978). Carlioz H, Vogt JC, Barba L, et al. *J Pediatr Orthop* 1984;4:153-161.

Reviews surgical treatment of slipped epiphysis. Covers in situ pinning, various osteotomies, and a large experience with the Dunn operation.

Cuneiform osteotomy in the treatment of slipped capital femoral epiphysis. Pearl AJ, Woodward B, Kelly RP. *J Bone Joint Surg* 1961;43A:947-954.

Poor results were reported in 35% of cases. Refinements in surgical technique were suggested to reduce the incidence of avascular necrosis and nonunion. (Editor's note: Despite the efforts of numerous skilled operators, the incidence of complications associated with femoral neck osteotomy remains uncomfortably high.)

Osteotomy through the lesser trochanter for slipped capital femoral epiphysis. Southwick WO. *J Bone Joint Surg* 1967;49A:807-835.

Classic description of this difficult but useful procedure for correction of severe deformity associated with slipped capital femoral epiphysis.

Southwick osteotomy for severe chronic slipped capital femoral epiphysis: Results and complications. Salvati EA, Robinson JH Jr, O'Down TJ. *J Bone Joint Surg* 1980;62A:561-570.

This osteotomy gave good correction of the deformity but is a major surgical procedure that should be recommended only for severe, chronic slips.

Complications

The problem of evaluating in situ pinning of slipped capital femoral epiphysis: An experimental model and a review of 63 consecutive cases. Lehman WB, Menche D, Grant A, et al. *J Pediatr Orthop* 1984;4:297-303.

Review of 63 hips (in 49 patients) revealed 36.8% incidence of unsuspected pin penetration. Four types of experimental models representing different degrees of severity of slipped capital femoral epiphysis were designed and manufactured in the bioengineering laboratory. In situ pinning was performed on each model. They found that conventional radiographs were not reliable in assessing pin penetration, but fluoroscopic analysis provided verifiable correlation.

Chondrolysis complicating slipped capital femoral epiphysis. Ingram AJ, Clarke MS, Clarke CS Jr, et al. *Clin Orthop* 1982;165:99-109.
A review of 329 patients with slipped capital femoral epiphysis treated at the Campbell Clinic revealed 79 cases of acute chondrolysis. The complication was more common in females, blacks, acute-on-chronic slips, open reduction, proximal femoral osteotomies, and when the joint had been penetrated by an internal fixation device. Biopsy revealed an apparent self-perpetuating synovitis.

Slipped capital femoral epiphysis: Long-term follow-up study of one hundred and twenty-one patients. Boyer DW, Mickelson MR, Ponseti IV. *J Bone Joint Surg* 1981;63A:85-95.
Results were better after in situ fixation than after surgical and manipulative treatment. Twelve of 13 acute slips that were reduced demonstrated avascular necrosis in three and good results in nine.

Complications after cuneiform osteotomy for moderately or severely slipped capital femoral epiphysis. Gage JR, Sundberg AB, Nolan DR, et al. *J Bone Joint Surg* 1978;60A:157-165.
The high incidence of severe complications after wedge osteotomies of the femoral neck led to abandonment of the procedure. The authors recommend base of neck osteotomy as the better alternative for severe slipped capital femoral epiphysis.

Hip: Other Conditions

Congenital Coxa Vara

The hip. MacEwen GD, Ramsey PL. In Lovell WW, Winter RB (eds): *Pediatric Orthopaedics*. Philadelphia, JB Lippincott, 1978, vol 2, pp 721-803.
Reviews the clinical features, roentgenographic features, prognosis, and treatment of congenital coxa vara.

Congenital coxa vara: A retrospective review. Weinstein JN, Kuo KN, Millar EA. *J Pediatr Orthop* 1984;4:70-77.
A review of 42 cases. Hilgenreiner's angle is used as a means of determining the amount of surgical correction.

Infantile coxa vara. Pavlov H, Goldman AB, Freiberger RH. *Radiology* 1980;135;631-640.
A good review of radiologic features and differential diagnosis.

Observations on infantile coxa vara. Blockey NJ. *J Bone Joint Surg* 1969;51B:106-111.

> A brief discussion of congenital and infantile coxa vara. Concludes that infantile coxa vara is due either to severe trauma in normal bone or to shearing stress in abnormal femoral necks.

Treatment of coxa vara in children by means of a modified osteotomy. Borden J, Spencer GE Jr, Herndon CH. *J Bone Joint Surg* 1966;48A:1106-1110.

> A technique of subtrochanteric osteotomy to correct coxa vara using a blade plate gave good results in five patients and seven hips.

Dysgenesis of the proximal femur (coxa vara) and its surgical management. Amstutz HC, Wilson PD Jr. *J Bone Joint Surg* 1962;44A:1-24.

> Discusses the three distinct groups: congenital short femur with coxa vara, congenital bowed femur with coxa vara, and congenital coxa vara. Surgical treatment of coxa vara has three aims: correction of the deformity, promotion of ossification of the cartilaginous neck, and prevention of recurrence. Surgical management is further discussed.

On pseudarthrosis of the femoral neck in congenital coxa vara. Langenskiold F. *Acta Chir Scand* 1949;98:568-575.

> Of 18 cases of developmental coxa vara in adults, 11 developed pseudoarthrosis. Of these, five were treated with McMurray osteotomy, and six with the Brackett operation.

Synovitis of the Hip

The hip. MacEwen GD, Ramsey PL. In Lovell WW, Winter RB (eds): *Pediatric Orthopaedics*. Philadelphia, JB Lippincott, 1978, vol 2, pp 721-803.

> A textbook review of transient synovitis including etiology, clinical features, radiologic features, diagnosis, and treatment.

Bone scintigraphy of hip joint effusions in children. Kloiber R, Pavlosky W, Portner O, et al. *AJR* 1983;140:995-999.

> Thirty-eight children with acute onset of hip pain were studied by bone scintigraphy.

Transient synovitis of the hip in the child: Increased levels of proteoglycan fragments in joint fluid. Lohmander LS, Wingstrand H, Heinegård D. *J Orthop Res* 1988;6:420-424.

> The levels of proteoglycan antigen were measured in joint aspirates from the hips of children with transient synovitis, septic arthritis, Legg-Calvé-Perthes disease and congenital and traumatic dislocation. Significantly increased levels were found in children with transient synovitis and septic arthritis as compared with other conditions.

Transient synovitis of the hip: A virological investigation. Blockey NJ, Porter BB. *Br Med J* 1968;4:557-558.

Studies of 17 children with transient synovitis of the hip did not confirm the suggestion that it was caused by a viral infection. The authors conclude that minor trauma is more likely the cause.

The characterization of "transient synovitis of the hip" in children. Haueisen DC, Weiner DS, Weiner SD, et al. *J Pediatr Orthop* 1986;6:11-17.
This is a recent retrospective review of 497 cases of transient synovitis of the hip. Follow-up attempting to establish the ultimate diagnosis indicated that it was a recurrent problem in 19 patients.

Transient synovitis and Legg-Calvé-Perthes disease: A comparative study. Gledhill RB, McIntrye JM. *Can Med Assoc J* 1969;100:311-320.
Legg-Calvé-Perthes disease occurred in approximately the same age distribution as transient synovitis but had a male preponderance and a higher incidence of bilateral involvement. Approximately 1% began as a synovitis that was clinically and radiologically indistinguishable from transient synovitis.

Recurrences of transient synovitis of the hip. Illingworth CM. *Arch Dis Child* 1983;58:620-623.
An excellent recent review of transient synovitis of the hip.

The Knee

Walter B. Greene, MD

Normal Development of the Knee

The natural history of torsion and other factors influencing gait in childhood: A study of the angle of gait, tibial torsion, knee angle, hip rotation, and development of the arch in normal children. Engel GM, Staheli LT. *Clin Orthop* 1974;99:12-17.

> Clinical measurements in 160 normal children in 16 age groups. Genu valgum and genu varum were measured on clinical photographs.

The development of the tibiofemoral angle in children. Salenius P, Vankka E. *J Bone Joint Surg* 1975;57A:259-261.

> Radiographic analysis of the tibiofemoral angle in children at different ages. Similar to the study by Engel and Staheli, this study demonstrated that children are born with genu varum and progress to excessive genu valgum in the first few years of life. Changes in radiographic measurements in this study lagged behind clinical measurements described in the study by Engel and Staheli.

Development of the menisci of the human knee joint: Morphological changes and their potential role in childhood meniscal injury. Clark CR, Ogden JA. *J Bone Joint Surg* 1983;65A:538-547.

> The vascularity, histologic characteristics, and biochemical composition of the meniscus were studied in 109 fetuses (14-34 weeks of gestation) and 28 cadavers (3 months to 14 years of age). Vascularity decreased with growth and changes progressed from the central to the peripheral margin. The shape of the menisci was determined early in prenatal development. Growth of the meniscus was uniform and commensurate with tibial growth.

Blood supply of the knee joint: A microangiographic study in children and adults. Shim SS, Leung G. *Clin Orthop* 1986;208:119-125.

> Detailed studies of changes in the vascular supply of the knee joint in pediatric and adult cadavers.

Distal femoral epiphysis: Normal standards for thickness and application to bone dysplasias. Schlesinger AE, Poznanski AK, Pudlowski RM, et al. *Radiology* 1986;159:515-519.

> Ratios of the distal femoral epiphysis height to both the distal femoral metaphysis width and the distal femoral epiphysis width were ascertained on 640 radiographs of healthy children at different ages.

These serve as standards for comparison in evaluation of patients with possible skeletal dysplasias.

Radiology of postnatal skeletal development: IX. Proximal tibia and fibula. Ogden JA. *Skeletal Radiol* 1984;11:169-177.
Radiology of postnatal skeletal development: X. Patella and tibial tuberosity. Ogden JA. *Skeletal Radiol* 1984;11:246-257.

These two papers describe radiographic changes with growth and discuss possible clinical relevance.

Surgical anatomy of selected physes. Birch JG, Herring JA, Wenger DR. *J Pediatr Orthop* 1984;4:224-231.

The relationship of the physis to surrounding structures and surgical exposure of the growth plate for excision of a bony bar are described in detail.

Assessment of normal pediatric knee ligament laxity using the genucom. Baxter MP. *J Pediatr Orthop* 1988;8:546-550.

Normal knees in 232 children ranging in age between 7 and 14 years were objectively analyzed for anterior/posterior and varus/valgus laxity. Laxity decreased progressively with growth. Tighter ligaments were seen in children who were above the 50th percentile for height and weight. No significant difference was seen in boys versus girls or in the right versus the left knee.

Congenital Anterior Subluxation/Dislocation of the Knee and Congenital Absence of Anterior Cruciate Ligaments

The etiology and treatment of congenital dislocation of the knee. Katz MP, Grogono BJ, Soper KC. *J Bone Joint Surg* 1967;49B:112-120.

Report of operative findings and results in 5 knees with congenital dislocation in children treated at a relatively old age (4-9). Describes a higher incidence of absent anterior cruciate ligaments and articular surface changes.

Congenital hyperextension with anterior subluxation of the knee: Surgical treatment and long-term observations. Curtis BH, Fisher RL. *J Bone Joint Surg* 1969;51A:255-269.

Classic article describing the surgical correction of resistant congenital hyperextension deformities of the knee. Associated deformities included arthrogryposis (77%), dislocation of the hip (91%), and congenital foot deformities (77%). Surgical technique was a V-Y lengthening of the quadriceps tendon, release of the anterior capsule, and release of other structures as needed. Results were better when surgery was done at an early age.

Congenital dislocation of the knee. Nogi J, MacEwen GD. *J Pediatr Orthop* 1982;2:509-513.

> In 17 patients (27 knees) with congenital dislocation of the knee but no other neuromuscular syndrome, good results were obtained by early closed treatment in 14 patients (82%). Hip abnormalities, seen in 8 patients, included "tight" hip adductors at birth (1), bilateral congenital dysplasia of the hip (2), and mild residual acetabular dysplasia (5). The Pavlik harness can be used to treat both hip and knee problems.

Congenital dislocation of the knee. Johnson E, Audell R, Oppenheim WL. *J Pediatr Orthop* 1987;7:194-200.

> Seventeen patients with 23 congenital knee dislocations were reviewed at an average follow-up of 11 years. Associated findings included breech delivery (41%), congenital dysplasia of the hips (71%), clubfeet (41%), and vertical tali (18%). Technique of open and closed treatment is described. Authors note difficulty in using the Pavlik harness in patients with rigid knee deformity. They agree with Curtis and Fisher in treating foot and knee deformities before the hip.

Congenital dislocation of the knee. Bensahel H, Dal Monte A, Hjelmstedt A, et al. *J Pediatr Orthop* 1989;9:174-177.

> In this multi-center study from the European Pediatric Orthopaedic Society, 56 cases of congenital dislocation of the knee were reviewed. Cases associated with such systemic diseases as arthrogryposis or Larsen's syndrome were excluded. Twenty-four cases were successfully treated conservatively and 32 required surgery. Only 2 children had a poor result. Knee flexion was greater in those who had reconstructive surgery compared with patients corrected by non-surgical therapy.

Percutaneous quadriceps recession: A technique for management of congenital hyperextension deformities of the knee in the neonate. Roy DR, Crawford AH. *J Pediatr Orthop* 1989;9:717-719.

> The technique of percutaneous quadriceps recession for congenital hyperextension of the knee is described. The authors note that range of motion was similar to that achieved by open procedures. Average age at surgery was 18 days.

Missing cruciate ligament in congenital short femur. Johansson E, Aparisi T. *J Bone Joint Surg* 1983;65A:1109-1115.

> Six of 42 patients with congenital short femur were found to have absence of the anterior cruciate or both cruciate ligaments. The deficiency was associated with hypoplasia of the tibial spines. Osteoarthritis was not found.

Congenital absence of the anterior cruciate ligament: A common component of knee dysplasia. Thomas NP, Jackson AM, Aichroth PM. *J Bone Joint Surg* 1985;67B:572-575.

Describes clinical and radiologic features in 10 patients with congenital absence of anterior cruciate ligament. Menisci were typically normal but secondary bony abnormalities were frequent. This condition is associated with other, more easily recognized congenital abnormalities.

Subluxation of the knee as a complication of femoral lengthening by the Wagner technique. Jones DC, Moseley CF. *J Bone Joint Surg* 1985;67B:33-35.
Seven of 14 patients with congenital hypoplasia of the femur developed knee flexion contracture and posterior subluxation of the tibia while undergoing leg lengthening. Treatments included skeletal traction, surgery, and plaster immobilization.

Genu Varum, Genu Valgum, and Genu Recurvatum

Control of bone growth by epiphyseal stapling: A preliminary report. Blount WP, Clark GR. *J Bone Joint Surg* 1949;31A:464-478.
The classic.

Epiphyseal stapling for angular deformity at the knee. Zuege RC, Kempken TG, Blount WP. *J Bone Joint Surg* 1979;61A:320-329.
Sixty-four knees with genu valgum and 18 knees with genu varum were treated by epiphyseal stapling. The technique is simpler and safer than osteotomy. A rebound growth effect may be seen after staple removal in certain children. Because exaggerated physiologic deformities can correct spontaneously, operations in these cases should be delayed until skeletal age 11 in girls and 12 in boys.

Partial epiphysiodesis at the knee to correct angular deformity. Bowen JR, Leahey JL, Zhang ZH, et al. *Clin Orthop* 1985;198:184-190.
A method of hemi-epiphysiodesis for correction of genu valgum or genu varum is described and results reviewed in seven patients. Three patients demonstrated good results, two angular deformities corrected early, one procedure was done late, and one patient had unilateral complication. The authors have devised a table that should make timing of the procedure more precise.

Fracture of the proximal metaphysis of the tibia in children. Skak SV, Jensen TT, Poulsen TD. *Injury* 1987;18:149-156.
Forty consecutive fractures of the proximal tibia metaphysis in children were reviewed. Fracture patterns included 17 buckle, 15 greenstick, and eight complete fractures. Valgus deformity occurred in 15% of the greenstick and complete fractures, but did not happen after buckle fractures. Valgus deformity was more common in the young children.

Spontaneous improvement of post-traumatic tibia valga. Zionts LE, MacEwen GD. *J Bone Joint Surg* 1986;68:680-687.
Seven children with post-traumatic tibia valga were followed for an average of 39 months after injury. Adequate clinical correction occurred

spontaneously in six of the seven patients. Observation of this problem is recommended until early adolescence.

Dysplasia of the knee associated with the syndrome of thrombocytopenia and absent radius. Schoenecker PL, Cohn AK, Sedgwick WG, et al. *J Bone Joint Surg* 1984;66A:421-427.

> Genu varum of varying severity was seen in 18 of 21 patients with the syndrome of thrombocytopenia and absent radius. Associated knee problems included internal tibial torsion and patellar abnormalities (absent, hypoplastic, or dislocated). Deformities were often severe and tended to recur after surgery because of intra-articular dysplasia.

Valgus deformity following derotation osteotomy to correct medial femoral torsion. Fonseca AS, Bassett GS. *J Pediatr Orthop* 1988;8:295-299.

> Progressive genu valgum developed in two patients (14%) who underwent bilateral distal femoral derotation osteotomies for persistent femoral anteversion. The deformity occurred secondary to medial femoral overgrowth. Both patients required a second surgical procedure to correct the deformity.

Asymmetrical arrest of the proximal tibial physis and genu recurvatum deformity. Pappas AM, Anas P, Toczylowski HM Jr. *J Bone Joint Surg* 1984;66A:575-581.

> Six cases of premature asymmetric closure of the proximal tibia physis and resultant genu recurvatum deformity are described. Fourteen previously reported cases are also reviewed. No single etiological factor could be implicated as a cause of the physeal arrest. The deformity was satisfactorily treated by an opening wedge osteotomy through the proximal one third of the tibia.

Treatment of genu recurvatum by proximal tibial closing-wedge/anterior displacement osteotomy. Bowen JR, Morley DC, McInerny V, et al. *Clin Orthop* 1983;179:194-199.

> In 14 patients (17 knees), four different procedures were used to correct genu recurvatum secondary to premature closure of the anterior portion of the proximal tibial physis. The authors conclude that the closing-wedge/ anterior displacement osteotomy has more advantages than other procedures. Surgical technique is described.

Angular and torsional deformities of the lower limbs in children. Kling TF Jr, Hensinger RN. *Clin Orthop* 1983;176:136-147.

> A good review article of the presentation, differential diagnosis, and treatment of these conditions.

Complications of tibial osteotomy in children for genu varum or valgum: Evidence that neurological changes are due to ischemia. Steel HH, Sandrow RE, Sullivan PD. *J Bone Joint Surg* 1971;53A:1629-1635.

> This classic article focuses attention on the high rate of neurologic or vascular complications following high tibial osteotomies in children.

Complications occurred in eight of 27 patients. (Editor's note: Current knowledge about compartment syndrome has led many authors to recommend prophylactic subcutaneous anterior compartment fasciotomy when doing this procedure in children.)

Knee Flexion Contractures

Flexion contractures of the knee associated with popliteal webbing. Addison A, Webb PJ. *J Pediatr Orthop* 1983;3:376-379.
Describes two patients with knee-flexion contractures associated with multiple pterygium and three patients with knee-flexion contractures associated with popliteal pterygium. Distinguishing characteristics of each group are presented. All patients required surgery, and the technique is outlined.

Posterior capsulotomy for the treatment of severe flexion contractures of the knee. Heydarian K, Akbarnia BA, Jabalameli M, et al. *J Pediatr Orthop* 1984;4:700-704.
Twenty-nine patients (42 knees) with knee flexion contractures averaging 69 degrees were treated by posterior capsulotomy followed by traction and/or casting. Twenty-eight cases had poliomyelitis. Thirty-nine knees were corrected to less than 15 degrees of flexion and walking status was significantly improved. Complications included skin necrosis in 9, recurrence in 6, hypertension in 3, and peroneal nerve palsy in 1.

The knee in arthrogryposis. Thomas B, Schopler S, Wood W, et al. *Clin Orthop* 1985;194:87-92.
Surgical treatment was necessary for knee flexion contractures in 31 of 104 patients with arthrogryposis multiplex congenita. Operative procedures included hamstring and posterior capsular release, epiphysiodesis, distal femoral or proximal tibial osteotomy, arthrodesis, and knee disarticulation. The most useful surgical procedure in the growing child was posterior capsular release performed in conjunction with hamstring tenotomy. Recurrence was common but was particularly frequent in osteotomies performed before completion of growth.

Subluxation of the knee as a complication of femoral lengthening by the Wagner technique. Jones DC, Moseley CF. *J Bone Joint Surg* 1985;67B:33-35.
Seven of 14 patients with congenital hypoplasia of the femur developed knee flexion contracture and posterior subluxation of the tibia while undergoing leg lengthening. Treatments included skeletal traction, surgery, and plaster immobilization.

The management of musculoskeletal problems in hemophilia: Part III. Nonoperative management of hemophilic arthropathy and muscle hemorrhage. In Greene WB, Wilson FC (eds): American Academy of Orthopaedic Surgeons *Instructional Course Lectures, XXXII*. St.Louis, CV Mosby, 1983, pp 223-233.

The technique of Quengel casting for correcting posterior subluxation of the tibia and knee flexion contracture using a Quengel cast is described. In 16 patients the knee flexion contracture was decreased from an average of 43 degrees to 8 degrees.

Knee Extension Contractures

Pathogenesis of infantile quadriceps fibrosis and its correction by proximal release. Sengupta S. *J Pediatr Orthop* 1985;5:187-191.

Thirty-three children (52 knees) developed extension contractures secondary to repeated intramuscular drug therapy which led to muscle fibrosis and contractures. The authors advocate release of the contracted muscles through a limited subtrochanteric exposure.

Injection-induced contractures of the quadriceps in childhood: A comparison of proximal release and distal quadricepsplasty. Jackson AM, Hutton PA. *J Bone Joint Surg* 1985;67B:97-102.

The authors compared conservative, distal quadricepsplasty, and proximal release for treatment of 32 knee extension contractures associated with repeated intramuscular injections. Conservative therapy did not improve range of motion. None of the patients treated by proximal release had an extension lag, a problem present in 70% of those treated by distal quadricepsplasty.

Arthroscopy of the Knee

Arthroscopic treatment of septic knees in children. Skyhar MJ, Mubarak SJ. *J Pediatr Orthop* 1987;7:647-651.

Twenty children (average age 2.7 years) were treated for septic arthritis of the knee by either early arthroscopic lavage or early arthrotomy. Both groups had good results on final follow-up examination. Arthroscopy is recommended because these patients exhibited earlier functional recovery and minimal post-operative incisional scars.

Arthroscopy in acute septic knees: Management in pediatric patients. Stanitski CL, Harvell JC, Fu FH. *Clin Orthop* 1989;241:209-212.

The authors report 16 children (average age 12 years) whose septic knees were treated by arthroscopic evacuation, debridement, and irrigation. Foreign bodies were also removed through the arthroscope in four patients. No post-operative irrigation or drainage system was used. The procedure, characterized by low morbidity, aided rapid restoration of joint motion.

Arthroscopy of the knee in children. Morrissy RT, Eubanks RG, Park JP et al. *Clin Orthop* 1982;162:103-107.

A consecutive series of 32 children undergoing knee arthroscopy included 11 children 13 years of age or younger, and 21 from 14 to 17 years of age. In the pre-adolescent group there was a smaller percentage of correct diagnosis before arthroscopy (27% versus 61%). Arthroscopy (1) distinguished serious intra-articular damage from unrecognized internal derangements, (2) defined the cause of synovitis, and (3) provided diagnostic help in patients with persistent pain but no demonstrable knee pathology.

Diagnostic arthroscopy of the knee in children. Suman RK, Stother IG, Illingworth G. *J Bone Joint Surg* 1984;66B:535-537.

Clinical diagnosis and arthroscopic findings were compared in 72 symptomatic knees in 68 children between 2 and 17 years of age. The clinical diagnosis was accurate in 42% of knees in 20 children up to 13 years of age compared with 55% in the older age group. The most common misdiagnosis in the younger children was discoid lateral meniscus. In children over 13, it was torn medial meniscus. Possible unnecessary arthrotomy was avoided in 58% of knees in the younger group and in 31% in the older group.

The role of arthroscopy in children. Ziv I, Carroll NC. *J Pediatr Orthop* 1982;2:243-247.

Consecutive arthroscopic examinations in 156 children with knee complaints were reviewed. Overall, arthroscopy was found to be very useful in 31%, useful in 63%, and not helpful in 6%. Under the age of 12 the most common diagnosis was discoid lateral meniscus and trauma to the knee joint.

Arthroscopy of the knee in children. Bergström R, Gillquist J, Lysholm J, et al. *J Pediatr Orthop* 1984;4:542-545.

Seventy-one knee arthroscopies in children younger than 16 years of age were reviewed. Hemarthrosis was the presenting complaint in 30. Nineteen of these patients had injuries to the medial, lateral or cruciate ligaments, of whom 11 knees required surgical repair or reconstruction. Forty-one arthroscopies were done in patients for chronic problems. A clinical diagnosis of meniscus tear was correct in only 20%.

Osteochondritis Dissecans

Osteochondritis dissecans in children. Green WT, Banks HH. *J Bone Joint Surg* 1953;35A:26-47.

A classic report that recognized osteochondritis dissecans as a common lesion in children that could frequently be treated by closed means.

A diagnostic sign in osteochondritis dissecans of the knee. Wilson JN. *J Bone Joint Surg* 1967;49A:477-480.

The author describes the diagnostic maneuver, now known as Wilson's sign, that may be present in osteochondritis dissecans.

Osteochondritis dissecans and other lesions of the femoral condyles. Bradley J, Dandy DJ. *J Bone and Joint Surg* 1989;71B:518-522.

One hundred seventy-four lesions of the femoral condyles were evaluated and characterized at arthroscopy. Lesions were separated into categories of developing and late osteochondritis dissecans, acute and old osteochondral fractures, chondral separations, chondral flaps, and idiopathic osteonecrosis. Osteochondritis dissecans was seen only at the "classical" site on the medial femoral condyle. Developing osteocondritis dissecans, seen only in those less than 18 years of age, was recognized as an area of ossification that had developed separately from the main portion of the femoral epiphysis. Late osteochondritis dissecans, differentiated from osteochondral fractures by its shape, presented as a loose body.

Osteochondritis dissecans of the femoral condyles. Hughston JC, Hergenroeder PT, Courtenay BG. *J Bone Joint Surg* 1984;66A:1340-1348.

In this review of 83 patients (95 knees) with osteochondritis dissecans, the authors advocate only symptomatic restriction of activity and quadriceps-strengthening exercises for patients diagnosed before physeal closure who have no evidence of "functional" disability. Surgical treatment was primarily removal of the loose body, but when the osteochondral fragment was similar to the defect in the femoral condyle, the treatment was multiple Kirschner wire fixation. Long-term results indicated that better results were obtained by open reduction and internal fixation. (Editor's note: A very worthwhile study to read; however, results are sometimes difficult to interpret due to the grouping of patients.)

99m-Technetium phosphate compound joint scintigraphy in the management of juvenile osteochondritis dissecans of the femoral condyles. Cahill BR, Berg BC. *Am J Sports Med* 1983;11:329-335.

Eighteen patients from 9 to 17 years of age were studied with sequential bone scans. Typical progression was marked by increased uptake in the area of the osseous defect, increased avidity in the involved femoral condyle, increased avidity on the scan only in the area of the osseous defect, and, subsequently, a normal bone scan.

Osteochondritis dissecans of the posterior femoral condyle. Outerbridge RE. *Clin Orthop* 1983;175:121-129.

Massive osteochondritis dissecans of the weightbearing posterior surface of the distal femoral condyle was reported in 14 patients (16 knees). Onset of symptoms was typically before age 15. All patients were male and most were actively involved with athletic activities. Spontaneous healing was seen before the age of 15 years. A persistent osteochondral fragment after age 15 typically progressed to fragment separation.

Neuropathic osteonecrosis of the lateral femoral condyle in childhood: A report on four cases. Citron ND, Paterson FW, Jackson AM. *J Bone Joint Surg* 1986;68B:96-99.

Four children with a motor and sensory deficit in the affected limb developed spontaneous osteonecrosis affecting a large portion of the lateral femoral condyle. Valgus deformities of the lower extremity with repeated excessive loading of the lateral femoral condyle can produce these lesions in "neuropathic" extremities. Closed treatment was not successful.

Meniscus Lesions (Discoid Meniscus)

Discoid lateral meniscus of the knee joint: Nature, mechanism, and operative treatment. Kaplan EB. *J Bone Joint Surg* 1957;39A:77-87.
>A well-known anatomic and pathologic description of this condition. Kaplan advocated the importance of the posterior horn having (1) no posterior attachment to the tibia plateau and (2) the ligament of Wrisberg linking the discoid meniscus to the femoral condyle.

The discoid lateral-meniscus syndrome. Dickhaut SC, DeLee JC. *J Bone Joint Surg* 1982;64A:1068-1073.
>Ten of 12 patients with a complete type of discoid lateral meniscus (intact ligament attachments) were asymptomatic. These patients were older and were having arthroscopic examinations for other pathology. Six patients averaging 14 years of age had a snapping knee secondary to a Wrisberg-ligament type of discoid lateral meniscus. Four of these six patients had a vertical tear in the posterior horn of the discoid meniscus.

Lateral discoid menisci in children. Bellier G, Dupont JY, Larrain M, et al. *Arthroscopy* 1989;5:52-56.
>Loss of physiologic hyperextension of the knee with a history of the snapping knee syndrome suggests the diagnosis of a torn lateral discoid meniscus. Arthroscopic meniscectomy was used in 19 knees (average age 10.5 years), with excellent results reported in 18 cases.

Arthroscopic meniscectomy for discoid lateral meniscus in children. Hayashi LK, Yamaga H, Ida K, et al. *J Bone Joint Surg* 1988;70A:1495-1500.
>Reviews 56 children less than 15 years of age with symptomatic lateral discoid meniscus. None of the affected knees were of the Wrisberg-ligament type. Because of the unique anatomy of the discoid meniscus, the authors advocate a partial meniscectomy with preservation of a rim limited to 6 mm for complete lesions and 8 mm for incomplete lesions.

Meniscus Lesions (Meniscus Tears)

Meniscal lesions in children and adolescents: A review of the pathology and clinical presentation. King AG. *Injury* 1983;15:105-108.
>Reviews 56 arthrotomies in children suspected of having meniscal lesions. In children, an accurate history, physical examination,

prolonged observation, and even direct inspection at arthrotomy may be unreliable in determining the true pathology.

Meniscectomy in children: A long-term follow-up study. Manzione M, Pizzutillo PD, Peoples AB, et al. *Am J Sports Med* 1983;11:111-115.
> Twenty children and adolescents with isolated meniscal tears were examined an average of 5.5 years after surgery. At follow-up exams, 60% had unsatisfactory results. Clinical results did not correlate with the site of meniscectomy, the type of meniscal tear, the severity of radiographic changes, or whether the meniscectomy was total or partial.

Late results after meniscectomy in children. Søballe K, Hansen AJ. *Injury* 1987;18:182-184.
> Seventy-five children were reviewed at an average 15 years after meniscectomy. Osteoarthritis was common in those with the longer follow-up times.

Knee Ligament Injuries

Prophylactic knee braces and injury to the lower extremity. Grace TG, Skipper BJ, Newberry JC, et al. *J Bone Joint Surg* 1988;70A:422-427.
> Three hundred thirty high school football players wearing prophylactic knee braces were compared to 250 athletes who did not wear braces. The group wearing single hinge braces had a significantly increased number of knee injuries. Participants wearing the double hinged braces had a higher number of knee injuries, but the difference was not significant. Injuries of the ankle and foot were more common in athletes who wore braces. These results question the efficacy of prophylactic knee braces.

Nonoperative management of isolated grade III collateral ligament injury in high school football players. Jones RE, Henley MB, Francis P. *Clin Orthop* 1986;213:137-140.
> Twenty-two of 24 high school football players achieved a stable knee and returned to competitive sports after closed treatment of a grade III injury of the medial collateral ligament. The authors emphasize the active rehabilitation program and controlled motion in a rehabilitation knee brace.

Poor results of anterior cruciate ligament repair in adolescence. Engebretsen L, Svenningsen S, Benum P. *Acta Orthop Scand* 1988;59:684-686.
> Eight adolescents were followed for three to eight years after primary suture of a midsubstance rupture of the anterior cruciate ligament. Only three patients had good function, and five were unstable.

Anterior cruciate ligament injuries in the young athlete with open physes. McCarroll JR, Rettig AC, Shelbourne KD. *Am J Sports Med* 1988;16:44-47.

Forty patients under 14 years of age with open physes were treated for midsubstance tears of the anterior cruciate ligament. Non-surgical treatment was used in 16. Only seven of these patients returned to sports, and all experienced recurrent episodes of knee instability. Twenty-four patients underwent either an extra-articular or intra-articular reconstruction based on growth potential. All 24 of these patients returned to sports activities. The authors suggest a treatment plan based on the degree of instability, the presence or absence of meniscal tears, and the athletic desires of the patient and his/her family.

Tears of the anterior cruciate ligament in adolescents. Lipscomb AB, Anderson AF. *J Bone Joint Surg* 1986;68A:19-28.
> The authors report 16 excellent, seven good, and one fair result in athletes, 12 to 15 years old, who had surgical reconstruction of a torn anterior cruciate ligament, using the semitendinosus and gracilis tendons. All torn menisci should be repaired if possible. Limb-length discrepancy at completion of growth was significant in only one patient.

Ligament injuries associated with physeal fractures about the knee. Bertin KC, Goble EM. *Clin Orthop* 1983;177:188-195.
> Distal femoral physeal fractures demonstrated a 32% incidence of ligament instability at follow-up evaluation. For proximal tibial physeal fractures the incidence was 62%.

Fractures of the tibial spine in children: An evaluation of knee stability. Baxter MP, Wiley JJ. *J Bone Joint Surg* 1988;70:228-230.
> Forty-five patients with fractures of the tibial spine were evaluated three to ten years after injury. No patient complained of knee instability, but 51% had a measurable degree of cruciate ligament laxity. Collateral ligament instability was infrequently observed. No difference in anterior translations was found in fractures treated by closed versus open reduction.

Patellar Subluxation/Dislocation (Congenital and Habitual)

Congenital lateral dislocation of the patella. Green JP, Waugh W, Wood H. *J Bone Joint Surg* 1968;50B:285-289.
> Four cases are described. The authors emphasize the associated flexion contracture and the need for early treatment.

Congenital, irreducible, permanent lateral dislocation of the patella. Stanisavljevic S, Zemenick G, Miller D. *Clin Orthop* 1976;116:190-199.
> A comprehensive review of the literature. The authors describe a procedure that includes proximal realignment of the origin of the vastus lateralis, release of the vastus lateralis retinaculum, plication of the vastus medialis retinaculum, and rerouting of the lateral division of the patellar tendon. The procedure has been done in seven knees, including five patients with Down syndrome. No long-term results are reported.

Semitendinosus tenodesis for recurrent subluxation or dislocation of the patella. Hall JE, Micheli LJ, McManama GB Jr. *Clin Orthop* 1979;144:31-35.

> Describes the results of a proximal quadriceps realignment augmented by transfer of the semitendinosus tendon in 21 patients (26 knees). There were three congenitally dislocated patellae, and nine patients had extreme ligamentous laxity. The group with ligamentous laxity had 22% excellent and good results, compared with 85% excellent and good results in the other subgroups.

Instability of the patellofemoral joint in Down syndrome. Dugdale TW, Renshaw TS. *J Bone Joint Surg* 1986;68A:405-413.

> When 361 patients with Down syndrome were evaluated to determine the prevalence of patellofemoral joint instability, 70% of the joints were stable, 21.7% could be subluxated more than one-half of the patella width but were not dislocatable, the patella was dislocatable in 5.5%, in 1.9% the patella was dislocated but could be reduced manually, and in 0.9% the patella was dislocated and could not be reduced manually. Almost all patients with patellofemoral joint instability were able to walk, although their ambulation was compromised. More severe degrees of patellofemoral instability correlated with development of other bony deformities.

Treatment of patellofemoral instability in Down's syndrome. Mendez AA, Keret D, MacEwen GD. *Clin Orthop* 1988;234:148-158.

> In this review of 16 patients (26 knees) with Down's syndrome and dislocatable or dislocated patellae, the authors observed no correlation between the degree of patellofemoral instability and ambulatory status. Closed treatment maintained the ambulation status in two thirds of the knees characterized as having fair or good ambulation. Surgery initially improved ambulatory ability in 86% of patients who had a fair or poor preoperative ambulatory status, but did not correct deformities that subsequently resulted in degenerative arthritis.

Patellar instability in juvenile amputees. McIvor JB, Gillespie R. *J Pediatr Orthop* 1987;7:553-556.

> In 41 patients with either a Syme or below-knee amputation, 12 had patellofemoral malalignment problems. All symptomatic patients had patella alta, lateral subluxation, and hypoplastic patellae. Four patients were treated by extension of the prosthesis, and three had surgical procedures.

Habitual dislocation of the patella in flexion. Bergman NR, Williams PF. *J Bone Joint Surg* 1988;70B:415-419.

> Reviews 35 patients (43 affected knees) with habitual dislocation of the patella. The authors distinguish congenital dislocation, habitual dislocation, and recurrent dislocation. The physical sign of habitual dislocation is lateral dislocation of the patella each time the knee is flexed. Pathoanatomy included well-defined bands or contractures within the vastus lateralis in 72%, the rectus femoris in 42%, the vastus

intermedius in 16%, and an abnormal attachment of the iliotibial tract in 58%. The surgical procedures included proximal releases and realignment. Of 12 knees that redislocated after surgery, 10 underwent a successful repeat quadricepsplasty.

Recurrent Patellar Subluxation/Dislocation

Acute dislocation of the patella in children: The natural history. McManus F, Rang M, Heslin DJ. *Clin Orthop* 1979;139:88-91.
> Reviews 33 children with acute dislocation of the patella. Osteochondral fragments required early surgery in three patients. Of the remaining 30, 5 (17%) required surgery for redislocation, but another group of 11 complained of a feeling of insecurity in the knee. Most patients had radiographic signs of patellofemoral dysplasia.

Treatment of acute patellar dislocation. Cash JD, Hughston JC. *Am J Sports Med* 1988;16:244-249.
> Reviews 100 patients (103 knees) to determine the effectiveness of treatment for an initial acute patellar dislocation. Based on an examination of the unaffected knee, patients were divided into group I (congenital abnormality of the extensor mechanism, n=69) or group II (no clinically perceptible congenital predisposition to dislocation, n=34). Closed treatment resulted in a 52% incidence of good or excellent results in group I and 75% in group II. Recurrent dislocation was more frequent in patients whose initial dislocation occurred before age 15.

The tangential x-ray investigation of the patellofemoral joint: X-ray technique, diagnostic criteria and their interpretation. Laurin CA, Dussault R, Levesque HP. *Clin Orthop* 1979;144:16-26.
> The authors describe a radiographic technique for visualizing the patellofemoral joint in a position that simulates patellofemoral malalignment problems. The principles of their technique are fundamentally sound and influenced the next two reports.

The evaluation of patellofemoral pain using computerized tomography: A preliminary study. Schutzer SF, Ramsby GR, Fulkerson JP. *Clin Orthop* 1986;204:286-293.
> Twenty patients with persistent patellofemoral pain and 10 asymptomatic volunteers had multiple mid-patella computed tomographic images obtained between 0 and 40 degrees of knee flexion. Eleven patients had high-congruence angles consistent with lateralized patella. With progressive knee flexion to 30 degrees, all but one of these patients reduced into the trochlea.

Subluxation of the patella: Computed tomography analysis of patellofemoral congruence. Inoue M, Shino K, Hirose H, et al. *J Bone Joint Surg* 1988;70A:1331-1337.

Compares 50 patients with a clinical diagnosis of patellar instability with 30 control subjects, using radiographs of the patellofemoral joint made with the knee in 30 and 45 degrees of flexion as well as computed tomography scans made with the knee in full extension. The study indicated that patellar subluxation can be detected more accurately by using computed tomography with the knee in full extension than by using conventional radiographic studies.

Current concepts review: Patellar pain. Insall J. *J Bone Joint Surg* 1982;64A:147-152.

This excellent review by a recognized expert outlines the cause, clinical presentation, diagnostic signs, and treatment of patellar disorders. Cautions against overuse of lateral release for patellar malalignment syndromes. Assuming proper selection, this procedure is effective in half of the knees, whereas a proximal realignment with advancement of the vastus medialis and extensive lateral release will provide good or excellent results in 90%.

Medial subluxation of the patella as a complication of lateral retinacular release. Hughston JC, Deese M. *Am J Sports Med* 1988;16:383-388.

In 30 patients referred to the authors following an arthroscopic lateral retinacular release, a disabling medial subluxation of the patella developed. Anterior knee pain was the only reported preoperative symptom in 14 knees. Sixteen knees had a preoperative diagnosis of lateral patellar subluxation on the basis of a positive apprehension sign only. Computed tomographic scan evaluation of three patients demonstrated severe atrophy and retraction of the vastus lateralis.

Patellar pain and incongruence. II: Clinical application. Insall JN, Aglietti P, Tria AJ Jr. *Clin Orthop* 1983;176:225-232.

Good or excellent results were found in 68 knees (91%) treated by a proximal realignment procedure. Authors outline the surgical technique and emphasize that their procedure is a quadricepsplasty rather than a medial imbrication and lateral retinacular release. A smaller percentage of good or excellent results were seen with more severe chondromalacia (fibrillations and erosions). There was little correlation between the severity of the cartilage lesions and the patients' pain.

Lateral release and proximal realignment for patellar subluxation and dislocation: A long-term follow-up. Scuderi G, Cuomo F, Scott WN. *J Bone Joint Surg* 1988;70A:856-861.

Fifty-two patients (60 knees) with either recurrent patellar subluxation or recurrent patellar dislocation were treated by a proximal realigment procedure. Good or excellent results were found in 81%. Better results were seen in patients less than 20 years of age and in males. The degree of chondromalacia did not seem to affect the overall results, but knees that needed a re-operation had progressed to severe patellofemoral osteoarthritis.

Patellar Problems, Other

Sinding-Larsen-Johansson disease: Its etiology and natural history. Medlar RC, Lyne ED. *J Bone Joint Surg* 1978;60A:1113-1116.

> Describes eight patients ranging from 10 to 13 years of age, who presented with pain at the inferior pole of the patella and had associated traction apophysitis of the inferior pole of the patella. Symptomatic treatment is recommended because this disease, like Osgood-Schlatter's disease, has a self-limited course.

Fragmentation of the proximal pole of the patella: Another manifestation of juvenile traction osteochondritis? Batten J, Menelaus MB. *J Bone Joint Surg* 1985;67B:249-251.

> Six boys, 10 and 11 years of age, were noted to have fragmentation of the proximal patella. Four patients had no symptoms referrable to the patella. The authors suggest that the fragmentation is secondary to a traction osteochondritis.

The natural history of anterior knee pain in adolescents. Sandow MJ, Goodfellow JW. *J Bone Joint Surg* 1985;67B36-38.

> Fifty-four females between 10 and 20 years of age with anterior knee pain had no evident meniscal or ligamentous pathology on clinical exam. In follow-up questionnaire, analyzed at two to 17 years after initial presentation, 95% continued to experience some pain, but the pain was worse in only 13%. In 46%, pain had diminished. Pain was felt about once a week or less frequently by 82%. There was no restriction of sports activities in 48%, but 17% had knee pain that severely restricted sporting activities. The authors recommend a policy of non-intervention for anterior knee pain in adolescence if there is no objective evidence of pathology.

Mechanical factors in the incidence of knee pain in adolescents and young adults. Fairbank JC, Pynsent PB, van-Poortvliet JA, et al. *J Bone and Joint Surg* 1984;66B:685-693.

> Evaluates 446 adolescents at a comprehensive school for measurements of joint mobility, lower-limb morphology, and knee pain. Joint laxity, the Q-angle, genu valgum, and anteversion of the femoral neck were not significantly different in those pupils with and those without anterior knee pain. The group with knee pain enjoyed sporting activities significantly more than their symptom-free contemporaries. The authors concluded that chronic overloading, rather than faulty mechanics, is the dominant factor in the etiology of anterior knee pain in adolescents.

Lateral facet syndrome of the patella: Lateral restraint analysis and use of lateral resection. Johnson RP. *Clin Orthop* 1989;238:148-158.

> Thirty-four patients (38 knees) had surgical treatment for lateral facet syndrome that did not respond to conservative therapy. Pre-operative evaluation demonstrated lateral patellofemoral joint line tenderness (95%), tenderness over the tendon of the vastus lateralis oblique (87%),

a positive medial apprehension test (76%), and marked resistance to passive medial patella displacement with the knee flexed to 30 degrees (63%). Surgery included division and resection of the vastus lateralis oblique tendon, the lateral retinaculum, and the anterior fibers of the iliotibial tract. With a minimum follow-up period of 2 years, 87% demonstrated relief of patellar pain and had returned to normal activities.

An electron microscopic study of early pathology in chondromalacia of the patella. Ohno O, Naito J, Iguchi T, et al. *J Bone Joint Surg* 1989;70A:883-899.

Ultrastructural observations on specimens from young patients who had chondromalacia were compatible with a pathogenesis resulting from mechanical overload.

Popliteal Cyst

Popliteal cysts in children: The case against surgery. Dinham JM. *J Bone Joint Surg* 1975;57B:69-71.

In 70 untreated popliteal cysts, 51 resolved spontaneously during a mean period of 1.7 years. By contrast, 21 of 50 cysts treated surgically recurred in a mean period of 0.6 years.

Infantile Tibia Vara

Tibia vara: Osteochondrosis deformans tibiae. Blount WP. *J Bone Joint Surg* 1937;19:1-29.

The classic.

Tibia vara (osteochondrosis deformans tibiae): A survey of seventy-one cases. Langenskiöld A, Riska EB. *J Bone Joint Surg* 1964;46A:1405-1420.

The classification described in this article has become standard, but subsequent papers have questioned whether the authors' recommendations for time of treatment can be used with the typical child in the United States who has infantile tibia vara.

A biomechanical analysis of the etiology of tibia vara. Cook SD, Lavernia CJ, Burke SW, et al. *J Pediatr Orthop* 1983;3:449-454.

Finite element analysis of the proximal tibia was used to calculate the stresses occurring in the physis during one-legged stance in 2- and 5-year-old children. Increasing varus resulted in increasing compressive stress in the medial aspect of the tibial physis. The compressive stress was 7 times normal at 30 degrees of varus. Changes were more marked in the obese child and in the 5 year old. The data supports the hypothesis that Blount's disease results from physical phenomena altering growth in the proximal tibial epiphysis.

Physiological bowing and tibia vara: The metaphyseal-diaphyseal angle in the measurement of bowleg deformities. Levine AM, Drennan JC. *J Bone Joint Surg* 1982;64A:1158-1163.

> The metaphyseal-diaphyseal angle allows differentiation of physiologic bowing versus infantile tibia vara. In 58 knees with a metaphyseal-diaphyseal angle of 11 degrees or less, only three had radiographic changes of infantile tibia vara. By contrast, in 29 of 30 knees with a metaphyseal-diaphyseal angle of 12 degrees or more, the radiographic changes of infantile tibia vara were either present or developed.

Radiographic measurement of infantile tibia vara. Foreman KA, Robertson WW Jr. *J Pediatr Orthop* 1985;5:452-455.

> The metaphyseal-diaphyseal angle and metaphyseal-metaphyseal angle were found to be reproducible in assessing bowleg deformities. The metaphyseal-metaphyseal angle became consistently larger with more severe varus, suggesting that abnormal growth in the distal tibial physis was also present with severe bowleg deformity.

Blount's disease: A retrospective review and recommendations for treatment. Schoenecker PL, Meade WC, Pierron RL, et al. *J Pediatr Orthop* 1985;5:181-186.

> Thirty-two patients (52 knees) were evaluated for treatment of Blount's disease. Five of six extremities having early brace treatment were rated good. Surgical treatment before 5 years of age was rated good in 83%, but in older children repeat osteotomies were frequently necessary, and only 38% of the extremities achieved a good rating. The authors recommend combining proximal valgus-correcting tibial osteotomy with other procedures for children of 5 years or older.

Infantile tibia vara: Factors affecting outcome following proximal tibial osteotomy. Ferriter P, Shapiro F. *J Pediatr Orthop* 1987;7:1-7.

> This retrospective review of 37 cases of infantile tibia vara demonstrated that 57% required one to four additional osteotomies. Factors associated with recurrent deformity included massive obesity, Langenskiöld grade III or greater lesion, and initial osteotomy after 4.5 years of age.

Infantile tibia vara. Loder RT, Johnston CE II. *J Pediatr Orthop* 1987;7:639-646.

> Evaluates 73 cases (48 patients) of infantile tibia vara. Brace therapy was successful in one half of the extremities. No difference was found between the brace failure and success groups in regard to age, time of brace treatment, or initial deformity. The initial tibial osteotomy provided good results in 75% when the surgery was performed before 4 years of age, but in only 32% of those 4 years or older. The authors question the accuracy of Langenskiöld's estimate of prognosis.

Tibia vara: A critical review. Langenskiöld A. *Clin Orthop* 1989;246:195-207.

The author reviews the presentation, treatment and expected results for
(1) infantile tibia vara, (2) adolescent tibia vara, and (3) late onset tibia
vara. The author stresses that his radiographic classification system
represents developmental roentgenographic changes rather than
depictions of prognosis or results of treatment. The author, who has
had a minimal number of complications using a dome osteotomy,
describes technical aspects of this procedure.

Blount's disease after skeletal maturity. Hofmann A, Jones RE, Herring JA. *J
Bone Joint Surg* 1982;64A:1004-1009.
> Evaluates 19 knees in 12 patients aged 17 to 25. The age at initial
> proximal tibial osteotomy averaged 7.5 years (range four to 11 years).
> Twelve knees (63%) were symptomatic, with eight of the 12 showing
> early degenerative changes.

Late-Onset Tibia Vara and Adolescent Tibia Vara

Late-onset tibia vara: A comparative analysis. Thompson GH, Carter JR,
Smith CW. *J Pediatr Orthop* 1984;4:185-194.
> Reviews 11 children (16 knees) with delayed onset tibia vara. Six
> children had their onset between 6 and 9 years of age, and 5 at between
> 12 and 14 years of age. Fifteen knees were treated by proximal tibial
> valgus osteotomies. Males with juvenile onset type of tibia vara
> demonstrated a 50% rate of recurrent deformity.

The evolution and histopathology of adolescent tibia vara. Wenger DR,
Mickelson M, Maynard JA. *J Pediatr Orthop* 1984;4:78-88.
> Seven patients (nine knees) were reviewed to define clinical and
> radiographic characteristics. Typically these obese patients had
> maintained a mild degree of infantile physiologic genu varum that,
> concurrent with their adolescent growth spurt, demonstrated further
> progression. In 2 cases, histologic examination demonstrated fissuring
> and clefts in the physis as well as fibrovascular and cartilaginous repair
> tissue at the physeal-metaphyseal junction.

Clinical basis for a mechanical etiology in adolescent Blount's disease. Beskin
JL, Burke SW, Johnston CE II, et al. *Orthopedics* 1986;9:365-370.
> Clinical and radiographic characteristics of eight patients (ten knees) with
> late onset tibia vara were reviewed. Consistent clinical features included
> progressive varus during the adolescent growth spurt and gross obesity.
> Measurements of the physeal width of the proximal tibia and distal femur
> were consistent with adolescent tibia vara being caused by abnormal
> growth secondary to aberrant forces as predicted by Heuter-Volkman
> and Delpech's laws.

Late-onset tibia vara: A histopathologic analysis: A comparative evaluation with
infantile tibia vara and slipped capital femoral epiphysis. Carter JR, Leeson
MC, Thompson GH, et al. *J Pediatr Orthop* 1988;8:187-195.

Histopathologic and histochemical studies were performed on the entire physis of three patients with late-onset tibia vara. Disorganization and misalignment of the physeal zones were remarkably similar to those observed in both infantile tibia vara and slipped capital femoral epiphysis. The authors conclude that asymmetric compressive and shear forces acting across the proximal tibial physis caused the observed changes.

Osgood-Schlatter's Disease

Osgood-Schlatter's disease and tibial tuberosity development. Ogden JA, Southwick WO. *Clin Orthop* 1976;116:180-189.

Based on the development of the tibial tuberosity growth plate in fetuses, radiologic observations of the tibial tuberosity, and roentgenographic study in 53 patients with Osgood-Schlatter's disease, the authors conclude that Osgood-Schlatter's disease results from an inability of a developing secondary ossification center to withstand tensile forces, resulting in avulsion of segments of the ossification center, and eventual formation of heterotopic bone.

Does Osgood-Schlatter disease influence the position of the patella? Jakob RP, von Gumppenberg S, Engelhardt P. *J Bone Joint Surg* 1981;63B:579-582.

The Blackburn and Peel method was used to assess the position of the patella. A normal index of 0.80 was found in control knees, but the average index in the knees with Osgood-Schlatter's disease measured 1.01 (patella alta) in boys and 0.91 in girls. The index increased to 1.06 in boys with radiologic evidence of loose ossicles in the tibial tuberosity or the patellar tendon. This study supports the theory that Osgood-Schlatter's disease has a mechanical etiology and is a "traction apophysitis."

The so-called unresolved Osgood-Schlatter lesion: A concept based on fifteen surgically treated lesions. Mital MA, Matza RA, Cohen J. *J Bone Joint Surg* 1980;62A:732-739.

Of 151 knees treated for Osgood-Schlatter's disease, 15 had erosion of a distinct and separate ossicle at the proximal aspect of the tibial tubercle associated with persistent discomfort despite conservative therapy that averaged 3.8 years from the onset of symptoms to operation. (Editor's note: See several letters generated in response to this article in *J Bone Joint Surg* 1981;63A:170-171.)

Surgical treatment of Osgood-Schlatter's disease. Glynn MK, Regan BF. *J Pediatr Orthop* 1983;3:216-219.

In a series that compares two operations for Osgood-Schlatter's disease, a much higher incidence of excellent or good results were seen in the group treated by simple excision of "loose ossicles," compared with the group treated by drilling of the tibial tubercle with or without removal of the prominence.

Osgood-Schlatter's disease in adolescent athletes: Retrospective study of incidence and duration. Kujala UM, Kvist M, Heinonen O. *Am J Sports Med* 1985;13:236-241.

>Sixty-eight adolescent athletes were seen for Osgood-Schlatter's disease at an outpatient sports clinic. The average age at onset of symptoms was 13.1 years. Pain caused complete cessation of training for an average of 3.2 months, and the disease interfered with fully effective training for an average of 7.3 months. In a questionnaire given to 389 adolescent students, the incidence of Osgood-Schlatter's disease was 21.2% in those active in sports, but only 4.5% in those who were not active. A previous history of calcaneal apophysitis (Sever's disease) or a sibling with Osgood-Schlatter's disease was associated with a higher incidence of Osgood-Schlatter's disease.

Congenital Anterior Angulation and Pseudarthrosis of the Tibia

Pathology and natural history of congenital pseudarthrosis of the tibia. Boyd HB. *Clin Orthop* 1982;166:5-13.

>The most complete description of Boyd's classification system, the one most accepted. Type II, characterized by anterior bowing and hourglass constriction of the tibia present at birth, is most common and has the poorest prognosis.

Congenital pseudarthrosis of the tibia. Morrissy RT, Riseborough EJ, Hall JE. *J Bone Joint Surg* 1981;63B:367-375.

>Of 40 patients with congenital pseudarthrosis of the tibia, nine had good results, nine had fair results, eight had poor results, and 14 underwent amputation. No surgical procedure except the Farmer operation showed any clear superiority. Factors associated with poor results included considerable shortening, older children, and rapid resorption of the bone graft.

Congenital pseudarthrosis of the tibia: A long-term follow-up study. Murray HH, Lovell WW. *Clin Orthop* 1982;166:14-20.

>Of 25 skeletally mature patients, the results were satisfactory in eight (32%). The authors emphasize that many patients initially classified as satisfactory were lost to follow-up at their institution and had an amputation done elsewhere. The subsequent need for amputation was only discovered as a result of this study. A greater percentage of satisfactory results was obtained in those who presented with a fracture after 8 years of age and in those who were braced and never subsequently fractured.

Congenital pseudarthrosis of the tibia: Long-term follow-up study. Crossett LS, Beaty JH, Betz RR, et al. *Clin Orthop* 1989;245:16-18.

Twenty-five patients with congenital pseudarthrosis of the tibia were analyzed at an average age of 36 years. Results at skeletal maturity (with one exception) did not change at subsequent follow-up exams. Ten patients (40%) had good results with normal activity levels and no brace requirements.

The Syme amputation in patients with congenital pseudarthrosis of the tibia. Jacobsen ST, Crawford AH, Millar EA, et al. *J Bone Joint Surg* 1983;65A:533-537.

Eight patients with congenital pseudarthrosis of the tibia had a Syme amputation at an average age of 8.2 years. Subsequent prosthetic fitting allowed the child to engage in normal play activities. Though none of the pseudarthroses healed, the Syme amputation is recommended when necessary because it provides a longer stump than conventional amputations, better skin coverage, and more potential for further growth.

Congenital pseudarthrosis of the tibia: Treatment with pulsing electromagnetic fields. The international experience. Kort JS, Schink MM, Mitchell SN, et al. *Clin Orthop* 1982;165:124-137.

Ninety-two patients with congenital pseudarthrosis were treated using pulsating electromagnetic fields over an 8-year period. Excluding 10 lesions (11%) which healed with refracture, 48 lesions (59%) healed, 34 (41%) failed to heal. The success rate in 23 type I and 34 type II lesions was 77% and 76%, respectively. Surgery in association with this treatment did not improve results. The most important variable was radiographic morphology of the nonunion gap.

Free vascularised fibular graft in the treatment of congenital pseudarthrosis of the tibia. Pho RW, Levack B, Satku K, et al. *J Bone Joint Surg* 1985;67B:64-70.

Five cases of congenital pseudarthrosis of the tibia were successfully treated by free vascularized fibular grafts. This technique includes radical excision of abnormal bone and soft tissue around the pseudarthrosis and permits primary bone lengthening and correction of deformity.

Free vascularized fibular grafts in the treatment of congenital pseudarthrosis of the tibia. Minami A, Ogino T, Sakuma T, et al. *Microsurgery* 1987;8:111-116.

Five patients with congenital pseudarthrosis were treated by free vascularized fibular grafts. Follow-up averaged 3.3 years. Bony union was attained in three patients. Fractures after bony union were common.

Treatment of congenital pseudarthrosis with the Ilizarov technique. Fabry G, Lammens J, Van Melkebeek J, et al. *J Pediatr Orthop* 1988;8:67-70.

Three case reports with limited follow-up demonstrating bony union of a congenital pseudarthrosis of the tibia associated with neurofibromatosis.

Congenital pseudarthrosis of the tibia: Factors that affect results. Morrissy RT. *Clin Orthop* 1982;166:21-27.

> To provide guidelines for more effective use of amputation in the treatment of congenital pseudarthrosis of the tibia, the author proposes criteria based on a literature review and his own personal study. Factors associated with an unsatisfactory result include (1) dysplastic as opposed to cystic appearance of the tibia, (2) previous failures at bone graft procedures, (3) a response to grafting by rapid resorption of the graft material, and (4) shortening of the leg.

Congenital pseudarthrosis of the tibia. Paterson D. *Clin Orthop* 1989;247:44-54.

> An overview of treatment options for congenital pseudarthrosis of the tibia. Extensive reference list.

Congenital pseudarthrosis of the fibula. Dal Monte A, Donzelli O, Sudanese A, et al. *J Pediatr Orthop* 1987;7:14-18.

> Three cases of congenital pseudarthrosis of the fibula are reported. A review of these patients and the previous ones reported in the literature indicate that patients who have this condition should be braced during the childhood years and have correction of any valgus deformity deferred until puberty.

Congenital Posterior Angulation of the Tibia

Congenital posteromedial bowing of the tibia and fibula. Pappas AM. *J Pediatr Orthop* 1984;4:525-531.

> A study of patterns of growth and development in 33 patients with congenital posteromedial bowing of the tibia and fibula showed the bowing accompanied by shortening of the tibia and fibula, an initial calcaneovalgus deformity of the foot, and a decrease in ankle motion that does not improve with age. The greater the initial bowing, the greater the ultimate leg length discrepancy.

Posteromedial bowing of the tibia: Progression of discrepancy in leg lengths. Hofmann A, Wenger DR. *J Bone Joint Surg* 1981;63A:384-388.

> Of 13 children with posteromedial bowing of the tibia followed for a mean of four years, nine had a leg length discrepancy of more than 2.5 cm. There was usually a progression of the discrepancy, indicating the need for follow-up of these children. The severity of the leg-length discrepancy seems to be related to the degree of the curve. Epiphysiodesis may be required.

Congenital posteromedial bowing of the tibia. Yadav SS, Thomas S. *Acta Orthop Scand* 1980;51:311-313.

> Of six patients with congenital posteromedial bowing of the tibia, the deformity was corrected in five by serial casting. One severe case

required anterior soft-tissue release. Conservative treatment is advocated.

Congenital posterior angulation of the tibia with talipes calcaneus: A long-term report on 11 patients. Heyman CH, Herndon CH, Heiple KG. *J Bone Joint Surg* 1959;41A:476-488.

Congenital posterior angulation of the tibia: A clinical entity unrelated to congenital pseudarthrosis. Krida A. *Am J Surg* 1951;82:98-102.

The Foot and Ankle

G. Paul DeRosa, MD

Normal Feet

Measurements on radiographs of the foot in normal infants and children.
Vanderwilde R, Staheli LT, Chew DE, et al. *J Bone Joint Surg* 1988;70A:407-
415.
> Radiographs were made of feet of 74 normal infants and children from 6
> months to 127 months of age. Means and deviations were calculated for
> 11 clinically useful angles. These data provide a standard for the
> assessment of deformities in patients.

Clubfoot

Conservative treatment of the resistant recurrent clubfoot. Kite JH. *Clin Orthop*
1970;70:93-110.
> The conservative treatment of resistant clubfoot does not differ from
> treatment of untreated clubfoot. If previous treatment has not produced
> too many adhesions, recurrent clubfoot can usually be corrected by
> casts. If bones are fused in an abnormal position, another operation will
> be required. In treating any clubfoot, success depends on knowledge
> and patience.

The pathological anatomy of club foot. Irani RN, Sherman MS. *J Bone Joint
Surg* 1963;45A:45-52.
> There are no primary abnormalities of vessels, nerves, muscles, or
> tendon insertions in idiopathic clubfoot. Only the anterior part of the
> talus is abnormal, probably as a result of defective cartilaginous anlage
> derived from a primary germ-plasm defect.

Congenital club foot in the human fetus: A histological study. Ippolito E,
Ponseti IV. *J Bone Joint Surg* 1980;62A:8-22.
> Histologic study of five clubfeet and three normal feet revealed several
> abnormalities that indicated the possibility of a retracting fibrosis as the
> primary etiologic factor of the clubfoot deformity.

A histochemical study of muscle in club foot. Gray DH, Katz JM. *J Bone Joint
Surg* 1981;63B:417-423.
> A histochemical analysis of 103 biopsies from 62 patients with
> idiopathic clubfeet revealed no significant difference between the

diameter of muscle fibers taken from normal and from affected legs aged under six months. This indicates that wasting of calf muscles is caused by a reduction in the number of fibers rather than their size.

Genetic aspects of club foot. Cowell HR, Wein BK. *J Bone Joint Surg* 1980;62A:1381-1384.
Idiopathic talipes equinovarus is the result of a multifactorial inheritance system modified by environmental factors. Male risk is greater because of a lower gene threshold number.

Resistant congenital club foot: One-stage posteromedial release with internal fixation. A follow-up report of a fifteen-year experience. Turco VJ. *J Bone Joint Surg* 1979;61A:805-814.
Of 240 patients with clubfeet treated by the Turco procedure, results were excellent in 83.8%, fair in 10.7%, and failure in 5.3%. Best results were obtained in children treated between 1 and 2 years of age. Causes and preventions of fair and poor results, as well as modification of the original technique, are described.

Surgical correction of the resistant clubfoot: One-stage posteromedial release with internal fixation. A preliminary report. Turco VJ. *J Bone Joint Surg* 1971;53A:477-497.
Describes a one-stage surgical procedure for correction of resistant congenital clubfoot that evolved during the treatment of 58 feet in 41 patients over a 7.5-year period.

Surgical management of resistant congenital talipes equinovarus deformities. Thompson GH, Richardson AB, Westin GW. *J Bone Joint Surg* 1982;64A:652-665.
Surgery was performed for resistant congenital talipes equinovarus deformity in 164 children (244 feet) with a follow-up of 2 years or more. Of the 3 groups (according to type of surgery), those who had complete posteromedial and plantar release as the initial surgical procedure showed the best results (86% satisfactory).

Neonatal operative treatment of club foot: A preliminary report. Ryöppy S, Sairanen H. *J Bone Joint Surg* 1983;65B:320-325.
Sixty-seven patients with 94 resistant club feet were treated surgically as soon after birth as all other postnatal problems could be excluded, the mean age being 12 days. No treatment was attempted before operation. After minimum follow-up of two years (mean 4.4 years) 90% were satisfactory with primary treatment, although nine feet required one or more additional operations. Of the 10% with unsatisfactory results, all but one became satisfactory following secondary treatment.

Long-term results of early surgical release in club feet. Hutchins PM, Foster BK, Paterson DC, et al. *J Bone Joint Surg* 1985;67B:791-799.
Reviews 175 patients with 252 clubfeet treated by early posterior release, with an average follow-up of nearly 16 years. Eighty-one

percent had satisfactory results. The eventual result depended on the type of bony deformity present at birth.

Long-term results of treatment of congenital club foot. Laaveg SJ, Ponseti IV. *J Bone Joint Surg* 1980;62A:23-31.
>Correction of the lateral talocalcaneal angle and improved movement of the foot and ankle can be obtained by proper manipulative and plaster-cast techniques and transfer of the anterior tibial tendon. Posteromedial release results in corrected lateral talocalcaneal angle, but may reduce motion of the foot and ankle.

Club foot: Observations on the surgical anatomy of dorsiflexion. Scott WA, Hosking SW, Catterall A. *J Bone Joint Surg* 1984;66B:71-76.
>A study of dorsiflexion in three normal feet and three feet with talipes equinovarus was made to determine anatomic features that might contribute to surgical failure. Dorsiflexion in normal feet was found to be essentially rotatory in nature, while a posterolateral tether was found in the club feet. Posterior and lateral release is advocated for surgical correction of the hindfoot in a child with a clubfoot deformity.

New concept of and approach to clubfoot treatment: Section I: Principles and morbid anatomy. McKay DW. *J Pediatr Orthop* 1982;2:347-356; Section II: Correction of the clubfoot. McKay DW. *J Pediatr Orthop* 1983;3:10-21; Section III: Evaluation and results. McKay DW. *J Pediatr Orthop* 1983;3:141-148.
>This three-section article describes a different concept of the pathoanatomy and treatment for clubfoot. Unrecognized internal rotation in the subtalar complex is the key principle. The operation is described in detail in Section II, and Section III includes an evaluation of 102 feet.

Complete subtalar release in club feet: Part I: A preliminary report. Simons GW. *J Bone Joint Surg* 1985;67A:1044-1055.; Part II: Comparison with less extensive procedures. Simons GW. *J Bone Joint Surg* 1985;67A:1056-1065.
>These two articles compare the complete subtalar release with less invasive procedures. The former reportedly produced a greater degree of correction and provided better foot-and-leg alignment.

The Cincinnati incision: A comprehensive approach for surgical procedures of the foot and ankle in childhood. Crawford AH, Marxen JL, Osterfeld DL. *J Bone Joint Surg* 1982;64A:1355-1358.
>Using this transverse incision at the level of the tibiotalar joint, a variety of operative procedures were performed in 99 patients (154 feet). The incision improves visualization of the medial, posterior, and lateral aspects of the foot and ankle, and at the same time results in excellent healing of the wound and an improved cosmetic appearance.

Plantar release in the correction of deformities of the foot in childhood. Sherman FC, Westin GW. *J Bone Joint Surg* 1981;63A:1382-1389.

Residual cavovarus deformities from clubfoot in 191 feet were treated by a plantar release followed by correction with serial cast applications. In children older than 6 years of age, with deformities from clubfoot, plantar release effectively alleviated residual cavus deformity.

Relapsed club foot. Evans D. *J Bone Joint Surg* 1961;43B:722-733.
A surgical procedure for correction of relapsed clubfoot is described, with evidence that the essential deformity of clubfoot is a medial displacement or rotation of the navicular bone on the talus.

A review of the Dillwyn Evans type collateral operation in severe club feet. Addison A, Fixsen JA, Lloyd-Roberts GC. *J Bone Joint Surg* 1983;65A:12-14.
The Dillwyn Evans operation was used in severe relapsed club feet to correct the sagittally breached or bean-shaped foot. Forty-five feet in 37 patients were followed for an average of 9 years and 9 months. Of these, 30 were considered satisfactory.

Transposition of the anterior tibial tendon in the treatment of recurrent congenital club-foot. Garceau GJ, Manning KR. *J Bone Joint Surg* 1947;29:1044-1048.
The frequent recurrence of the deformity in clubfoot may be caused by the faulty mechanism of the muscles everting and inverting the foot. This operation is intended to prevent rather than to correct the deformity. Satisfactory results were obtained in 83% of 110 feet treated by this procedure.

A radiographic study of skeletal deformities in treated clubfeet. Ponseti IV, El-Khoury GY, Ippolito E, et al. *Clin Orthop* 1981;160:30-42.
Of 32 patients with treated unilateral clubfoot deformity followed for 13 to 20 years, 28 had satisfactory functional results. Radiographic comparison of normal and clubfeet showed many clubfeet to have small, slightly flattened talar heads, decreased talocalcaneal angles, undersized or misshapen facets of the subtalar joint, and medially displaced naviculars.

Operative treatment of congenital idiopathic club foot. Cummings RJ, Lovell WW. *J Bone Joint Surg* 1988;70A:1108-1112.
Current concepts review.

Metatarsus Varus

The natural history of hooked forefoot. Rushforth GF. *J Bone Joint Surg* 1978;60B:530-532.
A prospective study was performed to determine the natural history of untreated idiopathic hooked forefoot using 130 feet of 83 children with a follow-up of 11 years. Of these feet, 86% were normal or only mildly deformed but fully mobile.

Abductor hallucis release in congenital metatarsus varus. Mitchell GP. *Int Orthop* 1980;3:299-304.

> In true congenital metatarsus varus, contraction or shortening of the abductor hallucis muscle and tendon is the primary deforming factor. Correction may be achieved either by division of the tendon, with release of the capsular attachment, or by complete release of the abductor hallucis muscle from its extensive attachment to bone and soft tissues.

Mobilization of the tarsometatarsal and intermetatarsal joints for the correction of resistant adduction of the fore part of the foot in congenital club-foot or congenital metatarsus varus. Heyman CH, Herndon CH, Strong JM. *J Bone Joint Surg* 1958;40A:299-310.

> A surgical procedure for correction of residual and resistant adduction deformity of the forefoot is described. Results were good or excellent in all 20 patients. In selected patients up to 8 years of age, this procedure appears preferable to more radical osteotomy, arthrodesis, or bone or joint resection.

The Heyman-Herndon tarsometatarsal capsulotomy for metatarsus adductus: Results in 48 feet. Stark JG, Johanson JE, Winter RB. *J Pediatr Orthop* 1987;7:305-310.

> A follow-up of 48 procedures revealed a 41% failure rate and 50% incidence of painful dorsal prominence. The authors question the benefit of this operation in treating forefoot adduction deformity.

Metatarsal osteotomy for the correction of adduction of the fore part of the foot in children. Berman A, Gartland JJ. *J Bone Joint Surg* 1971;53A:498-506.

> Metatarsal osteotomy is shown to be a satisfactory method of correcting persistent fixed adduction of the fore part of the foot, regardless of its cause, in a child 6 years of age or older. It may be combined with other surgical procedures to correct either valgus or varus deformity of the hind part of the foot.

Ball and socket ankle joint in metatarsus adductus varus (S-shaped or serpentine foot). Lloyd-Roberts GC, Clark RC. *J Bone Joint Surg* 1973;55B:193-196.

> Metatarsus adductus varus, an obstinate deformity that resists correction, is often caused by a ball-and-socket ankle joint. The rigid forefoot should be treated, but the relatively mobile hindfoot should be left undisturbed.

Skewfoot (forefoot adduction with heel valgus). Peterson HA. *J Pediatr Orthop* 1986;6:24-30.

> The author indicates that skewfoot must be differentiated from metatarsus adductus, metatarsus varus, and metatarsus adductovarus. Because the natural history of skewfoot is unknown, treatment alternatives must be carefully considered. If surgical procedures are undertaken, realignment of the tarsal bone should be supplemented by hindfoot bone stabilization.

Pes Cavus

A simple test for hindfoot flexibility in the cavovarus foot. Coleman SS, Chestnut WJ. *Clin Orthop* 1977;123:60-62.
> A simple test using a wooden block provides clinical information that can be documented and on which a rational therapeutic program can be based.

Operative treatment of pes cavus: Stripping of the os calcis. Steindler A. *Surg Gynecol Obstet* 1917;24:612-615.
> Steindler's description of his technique for stripping of the os calcis for treatment of pes cavus deformity.

Pes cavovarus: Review of a surgical approach using selective soft-tissue procedures. Paulos L, Coleman SS, Samuelson KM. *J Bone Joint Surg* 1980;62A:942-953.
> A standardized treatment program was used in 20 patients (27 feet) with employment of a radical plantar or plantar medial release as indicated, in combination with tendon transfers or osteotomy of the fore part of the foot, or both. A two-year follow-up revealed 85% acceptable results with no major complications.

Claw-foot deformity: Treatment by transfer of the long extensors into the metatarsals and fusion of the interphalangeal joints. Chuinard EG, Baskin M. *J Bone Joint Surg* 1973;55A:351-362.
> From a review of 37 feet in 19 patients with claw-foot deformity, four stages of the deformity were identified, as well as indications for specific surgical procedures when other treatment failed.

Osteotomy of the calcaneum for pes cavus. Dwyer FC. *J Bone Joint Surg* 1959;41B:80-86.
> This operation for treatment of pes cavus resulted in marked improvement in all 63 patients in whom it was performed. The operation consists of subcutaneous division of the contracted plantar fascia and correction of the varus deformity of the heel by removal of a wedge from the lateral aspect.

Tarsometatarsal truncated-wedge arthrodesis for pes cavus and equinovarus deformity of the fore part of the foot. Jahss MH. *J Bone Joint Surg* 1980;62A:713-722.
> Results in 34 patients in whom this procedure was performed showed advantages of improved stability, better correction, and wider surface area of bone contact with more certain union when compared with metatarsal arthrodesis.

Neuromuscular Foot Disorders

The split anterior tibial tendon transfer in the treatment of spastic varus hindfoot of childhood. Hoffer MM, Reiswig JA, Garrett AM, et al. *Orthop Clin North Am* 1974;5:31-38.
>   Describes a procedure that transfers half of the anterior tibialis tendon to the cuboid bone. Gait improved in 16 patients.

Split posterior tibial-tendon transfers in children with cerebral spastic paralysis and equinovarus deformity. Kling TF Jr, Kaufer H, Hensinger RN. *J Bone Joint Surg* 1985;67A:186-194.

Split posterior tibial-tendon transfer in spastic cerebral palsy. Green NE, Griffin PP, Shiavi R. *J Bone Joint Surg* 1983;65A:748-754.
>   These two articles use the principle of partial tendon transfer described by Hoffer for the anterior tibial tendon in spastic feet. This procedure is most useful when the anterior tibialis muscle is too weak for transfer and when the posterior tibial tendon is overactive.

Posterior tibial-tendon transfer in patients with cerebral palsy. Root L, Miller SR, Kirz P. *J Bone Joint Surg* 1987;69A:1133-1139.
>   A retrospective review of 57 posterior tibial tendon transfers through the interosseous membrane to the dorsum of the foot. For successful treatment, the foot had to correct passively to neutral and the heel cord had to be lengthened. Good or excellent results, observed in 27 of 30 feet in hemiplegics and 12 of 16 feet in diplegics, were found in only 2 of 11 feet in quadriplegic patients.

Posterior tibial tendon transfer: A review of the literature and analysis of 74 procedures. Miller GM, Hsu JD, Hoffer MM, et al. *J Pediatr Orthop* 1982;2:363-370.
>   Forty-three patients underwent anterior transfer of the posterior tibial tendon through the interosseous membranes over a 10-year period. By analysis and comparison with a review of the literature, guidelines were formed for the use of the procedure. Patients with Duchenne muscular dystrophy who have decreased gait function or brace fitting problems are ideal candidates for this procedure, with 26 of 28 satisfactory results.

The problems associated with flail feet in children and their treatment with orthoses. Fulford GE, Cairns TP. *J Bone Joint Surg* 1978;60B:93-95.
>   Problems in 53 children with flail feet due to myelomeningocele were overcome by fitting them with below-knee orthoses, which provide maximum stability and yet allow normal walking. Biomechanical principles and development of the orthoses are discussed.

The management of deformity and paralysis of the foot in myelomeningocele. Sharrard WJW, Grosfield I. *J Bone Joint Surg* 1968;50B:456-465.
>   Deformities of the foot in children with myelomeningocele are described and classified. In 241 feet, 433 operations were performed, with

successful correction of deformity in 81%. Describes the management of individual deformities and analyzes the causes of failure.

Operative treatment of the foot deformity in Charcot-Marie-Tooth disease. Karlholm S, Nilsonne U. *Acta Orthop Scand* 1968;39:101-106.
   The typical foot deformity in Charcot-Marie-Tooth disease consists of an equino-varus-excavatus position. This deformity can be treated by soft-tissue surgery alone, using the technique described. Prognosis depends not only on the results of surgical correction, but also upon inherent progressiveness of the muscular atrophies.

The role of foot surgery in progressive neuromuscular disorders in children. Levitt RL, Canale ST, Cooke AJ Jr, et al. *J Bone Joint Surg* 1973;55A:1396-1410.
   Long-term evaluation, following surgery to correct foot deformities, of 15 children with Charcot-Marie-Tooth disease or Friedreich's ataxia. Soft-tissue procedures and bone procedures by themselves, excluding triple arthrodesis, did not stand the test of time. The one indication for their use was as part of a staged plan of treatment.

Long-term results of triple arthrodesis in Charcot-Marie-Tooth disease. Wetmore RS, Drennan JC. *J Bone Joint Surg* 1989;71A:417-422.
   Evaluation of 16 patients with Charcot-Marie-Tooth disease, who had 30 triple arthrodeses. Average length of follow-up was 21 years. Of the 30 feet, two had excellent results, five good, nine fair, and 14 poor. Concludes that a triple arthrodesis should be considered only as a salvage procedure in patients with progressive peripheral neuropathy and that it should be limited to those with severe, rigid deformity.

The role of subtalar fusion in the treatment of valgus deformities of the feet. Grice DS. In Reynolds FC (ed): American Academy of Orthopaedic Surgeons *Instructional Course Lectures, XVI.* St. Louis, CV Mosby, 1959, pp 127-150.
   Fusion of the subtalar joint with bone grafts is a simple procedure that is useful in a variety of foot deformities. It is particularly well adapted to stabilization of flail foot and correction of valgus foot. When used appropriately and well performed, it is usually a definitive procedure.

Batchelor's extra-articular subtalar arthrodesis: A report on sixty-four procedures in patients with poliomyelitic deformities. Hsu LC, O'Brien JP, Yau AC, et al. *J Bone Joint Surg* 1976;58A:243-247.
   Early results were poor because of inexperience with the technique and poor selection of patients. The incidence of nonunion, which was high compared with other series, was attributed to more advanced age of patients (average 9.9 years). A common cause of nonunion was tightness of the heel cord.

A clinical study of the Batchelor subtalar arthrodesis. Gross RH. *J Bone Joint Surg* 1976;58A:343-349.

Results of subtalar arthrodesis in 34 feet in 22 patients showed a pseudarthrosis rate of 41%, considerably higher than that reported for the Grice extra-articular arthrodesis. Two factors seemed to be related to the high incidence of pseudarthrosis; the parallelism of the axis of the graft to the subtalar joint and the cortical nature of the graft.

New operation of drop-foot. Lambrinudi C. *Brit J Surg* 1927;15:193-200.
Lambrinudi describes his procedure for paralytic equinus as being able to control drop-foot even though the gastrocnemius is active and powerful. The procedure also permits range of motion at the ankle joint.

Long-term results following Lambrinudi arthrodesis. Bernau A. *J Bone Joint Surg* 1977;59A:473-479.
Results after Lambrinudi arthrodesis in 50 feet (40 patients) were good in 20, fair in 27, and failed in 3. Most of the patients had post-poliomyelitic paralysis. An extensive review of the literature provides indications and contraindications for the procedure.

Triple arthrodesis by inlay grafting: A method suitable for the undeformed or valgus foot. Williams PF, Menelaus MB. *J Bone Joint Surg* 1977;59B:333-336.
Describes a method of triple arthrodesis applicable to the undeformed and valgus foot, as encountered in poliomyelitis, spastic flatfoot, cerebral palsy, and spina bifida. The procedure involves inlay of the subtalar and midtarsal joints. Failure of fusion of the midtarsal joint, the only significant complication, occurred in three of 85 feet.

Foot deformities secondary to gluteal injection in infancy. Bigos SJ, Coleman SS. *J Pediatr Orthop* 1984;4:560-563.
Six children developed foot deformities associated with sciatic nerve dysfunction apparently caused by gluteal intramuscular injection. Identification of muscle imbalance, as well as appropriate correction of the deformity before implementation of muscle balancing procedures, attained satisfactory plantigrade in 5 patients. The superolateral gluteal area between the crest of the ilium and the greater trochanter is recommended as the preferred site for intramuscular injection.

Tenodesis of flexor hallucis longus for paralytic clawing of the hallux in childhood. Sharrard WJ, Smith TW. *J Bone Joint Surg* 1976;58B:224-226.
Tenodesis of the flexor hallucis longus, performed in 17 feet in 13 children afflicted with paralytic clawing of the hallux, gave good results in 15 feet. Review of this technique suggests that flexor hallucis longus tenodesis is the method of choice for treating this abnormality in infants.

Paralytic Foot

Foot and ankle deformities in arthrogryposis multiplex congenita. Guidera KJ, Drennan JC. *Clin Orthop* 1985;194:93-98.

In fifty-one patients with arthrogryposis multiplex congenita followed for an average of 12 years, talipes equinovarus, the most common foot and ankle deformity, was best treated by talectomy. Congenital convex pes cavus was the second most common deformity, but no good solution for this deformity was found in this diagnostic group.

The management of the foot and ankle in arthrogryposis multiplex congenita. Drummond DS, Cruess RL. *J Bone Joint Surg* 1978;60B:96-99.
Reviews 66 deformities of the foot and ankle in 42 patients with arthrogryposis multiplex congenita. Intracapsular procedures proved more successful than those done adjacent to the joint, and capsulotomy or talectomy was best for children younger than 3 years. Triple arthrodesis was best for older children.

Talectomy: A long-term follow-up evaluation. Cooper RR, Capello W. *Clin Orthop* 1985;201:32-35.
In a 20-year follow-up on 26 talectomies of various etiologies, 24 of 26 had satisfactory results as defined by a stable, plantigrade foot. The procedure is indicated only for rigid, severely deformed feet.

Management of the resistant myelodysplastic or arthrogrypotic clubfoot with the Verebelyi-Ogston procedure. Spires TD, Gross RH, Low W, et al. *J Pediatr Orthop* 1984;4:705-710.
The Verebelyi-Ogston procedure, consisting of subchondral excision of the talus and cuboid, was used to treat resistant clubfeet secondary to myelomeningocele or arthrogryposis. Careful operative technique, meticulous casting, and prolonged orthotic support are essential for successful management. Uncertainties exist about long-term status of the articular surface.

Flatfoot

The longitudinal arch: A survey of eight hundred and eighty-two feet in normal children and adults. Staheli LT, Chew DE, Corbett M. *J Bone Joint Surg* 1987;69A:426-428.
The authors studied both feet of 441 normal subjects who were asymptomatic. They used a footprint and calculated the arch index--that is the width of the arch compared to the width of the heel--and plotted this for each age group.

Corrective shoes and inserts as treatment for flexible flatfoot in infants and children. Wenger DR, Mauldin D, Speck G, et al. *J Bone Joint Surg* 1989;71A:800-810.
The best prospective study of the effect of treating flexible flatfeet in neurologically normal children. Analysis of results was obtained by standard radiographs before treatment, during treatment, and at the most recent follow-up. There was no significant difference between the

controls and those treated with either corrective shoes, Helfet heel cups, or custom-molded plastic inserts.

Hypermobile flat-foot with short tendo achillis. Harris RI, Beath T. *J Bone Joint Surg* 1948;30A:116-140.
> Hypermobile flatfoot with a short Achilles tendon should be distinguished from other forms of flatfoot. The age of the patient and the severity of the lesion determine treatment. Mild cases are best treated conservatively; severe cases benefit from surgery.

The prehallux (accessory scaphoid) in its relation to flat-foot. Kidner FC. *J Bone Joint Surg* 1929;11:831-837.
> Discusses the relationship of the prehallux to flatfoot and describes a surgical procedure for removal of the prehallux.

Calcaneo-valgus deformity. Evans D. *J Bone Joint Surg* 1975;57B:270-278.
> In the normal foot, the medial and lateral columns are about equal in length. In talipes equinovarus, the lateral column is longer than the medial column; in calcaneovalgus, it is shorter. To equalize the length of the columns in calcaneovalgus deformity, cortical bone grafts taken from the tibia are inserted to elongate the anterior end of the calcaneus.

An operative method for correction of certain forms of flatfoot. Lowman CL. *JAMA* 1923;81:1500-1502.
> Classic description by Lowman of his procedure for resistant flatfoot.

Congenital Vertical Talus

Congenital vertical talus. Osmond-Clarke H. *J Bone Joint Surg* 1956;38B:334-341.
> Congenital vertical talus, if not treated successfully, leads to an ugly, painful foot in adolescence. The operation described reduces subluxation at the talonavicular and subtalar joints.

Problems in the recognition and treatment of congenital convex pes valgus. Herndon CH, Heyman CH. *J Bone Joint Surg* 1963;45A:413-429.
> Describes clinical and radiographic characteristics of congenital convex pes valgus. Notes surgical procedures and reports results in 26 feet.

Pathomechanics and treatment of congenital vertical talus. Coleman SS, Stelling FH III, Jarrett J. *Clin Orthop* 1970;70:62-72.
> This preliminary report of four cases reviews the pathomechanics of congenital vertical talus and demonstrates the value of combined closed and open surgical treatment.

The pathological anatomy of convex pes valgus. Drennan JC, Sharrard WJW. *J Bone Joint Surg* 1971;53B:455-461.

Presents the concept that a neuromuscular imbalance between the invertors and evertors of the foot causes convex pes valgus. Describes pathologic anatomy in a case of convex pes valgus in a patient with myelomeningocele.

Congenital vertical talus: Treatment by open reduction and navicular excision. Clark MW, D'Ambrosia RD, Ferguson AB. *J Bone Joint Surg* 1977;59A:816-824.

Sixteen feet in 12 patients with true congenital vertical talus were treated by excision of the navicular as an adjunct to open reduction. Follow-up at 2 to 15 years showed only one patient required further surgical treatment.

Congenital vertical talus: The Riley experience. DeRosa GP, Ahlfeld SK. *Foot Ankle* 1984;5:118-124.

Reviews ten feet with nonparalytic congenital vertical talus treated by peritalar open reduction and anterior tibiales transfer into the neck of the talus. Clinical and radiographic evaluation revealed three excellent, three good, and four fair results.

Surgical correction of congenital vertical talus under the age of 2 years. Seimon LP. *J Pediatr Orthop* 1987;7:405-411.

A one-stage, relatively simple approach is described for correction of congenital vertical talus. Seven patients (ten feet) had either excellent or good results.

Tarsal Coalition

Etiology of peroneal spastic flat foot. Harris RI, Beath T. *J Bone Joint Surg* 1948;30B:624-634.

This classic description of peroneal spastic flatfoot emphasizes the anomalies of the bones of the tarsus.

The painful foot in the child. Wilkins KE. In Bassett FH III (ed): American Academy of Orthopaedic Surgeons *Instructional Course Lectures, XXXVII.* Park Ridge, IL, American Academy of Orthopaedic Surgeons, 1988, pp 77-85.

An excellent review of conditions that cause painful feet in children.

Talocalcaneal coalition and new causes of peroneal spastic flatfoot. Cowell HR. *Clin Orthop* 1972;85:16-22.

This review of the abnormalities of the talocalcaneal joint demonstrates several causes for peroneal spastic flatfoot. Recognition of these abnormalities allows a rational approach to the treatment of peroneal spastic flatfoot. Conservative measures are indicated as primary treatment.

Rigid painful flatfoot secondary to tarsal coalition. Cowell HR, Elener V. *Clin Orthop* 1983;177:54-60.

Rigid flatfoot secondary to tarsal coalition requires proper clinical and radiographic evaluation, including axial (Harris) views and lateral tomography in addition to standard views. Symptomatic calcaneonavicular coalition without degenerative changes is treated by resecting the bar and inserting the extensor digitorum brevis. If degenerative changes are noted, triple arthrodesis is performed. For talocalcaneal coalition, triple arthrodesis is performed only if conservative treatment fails.

Tarsal coalitions and peroneal spastic flat foot: A review. Mosier KM, Asher M. *J Bone Joint Surg* 1984;66A:976-984.

Tarsal coalitions have been demonstrated in the fetus and result from failure of differentiation and segmentation of primitive mesenchyme. Nonoperative management should be considered before attempting surgical treatment of any symptomatic tarsal coalitions, especially if degenerative changes are present.

Surgical reconstruction for calcaneonavicular coalition: Evaluation of function and gait. Chambers RB, Cook TM, Cowell HR. *J Bone Joint Surg* 1982;64A:829-836.

Nineteen patients with 31 involved feet were analyzed three to 14 years after surgery. All had pain before surgery, but none did afterwards. Function correlated with subtalar motion and was normal when motion was good.

Symptomatic calcaneonavicular bars: The results 20 years after surgical excision. Inglis G, Buxton RA, Macnicol MF. *J Bone Joint Surg* 1986;68B:128-131.

Long-term follow-up evaluation of 11 patients with 16 involved feet that had excision of calcaneonavicular bars. Eleven of 16 (69%) had a good or excellent result. Of the five that failed, three were satisfactory after subsequent triple arthrodesis. The two that were treated by re-excision of the bar remained unsatisfactory. Beaking of the talus seen before surgery correlated with poor results.

Computerized tomography of talocalcaneal tarsal coalition: A clinical and anatomic study. Herzenberg JE, Goldner JL, Martinez S, et al. *Foot Ankle* 1986;6:273-288.

The authors studied 22 patients who had suspected peroneal spastic flatfoot. Computed tomography demonstrated bony and nonbony coalitions in 14 of the 22 patients studied. In the remaining 8 patients, computed tomography effectively ruled out the diagnosis of subtalar coalition. Computed tomography was superior to the other modalities for clearly identifying all aspects of the subtalar joint and the talocalcaneal joint coalitions.

Excision of symptomatic coalition of the middle facet of the talocalcaneal joint. Olney BW, Asher MA. *J Bone Joint Surg* 1987;69A:539-544.

Excision of a coalition involving the middle facet of the talocalcaneal joint and interposition of an autogenous fat graft was performed on ten feet (nine patients). Results were rated as five excellent, three good, one fair, and one poor. Incomplete resection was associated with the poor result. The procedure is superior to a triple arthrodesis.

Treatment of symptomatic talocalcaneal coalition. Scranton PE Jr. *J Bone Joint Surg* 1987;69A:533-539.

Fourteen feet had resection of the coalition when symptoms were not relieved by plaster cast immobilization. Indications for resection included failure of conservative treatment, a coalition that is less than one half the surface area of the talocalcaneal joint, and absence of degenerative changes in that joint. No patient had a poor result. Prerequisites for treatment also included absence of degenerative change and a coalition less than one half the surface area of the talocalcaneal joint.

Tibialis spastic varus foot with tarsal coalition. Simmons EH. *J Bone Joint Surg* 1965;47B:533-536.

Tarsal coalition often presents with the clinical picture of peroneal spastic flatfoot, but can present with a painful varus foot and spasm of the tibial muscles. Three cases of tibialis spastic varus foot had a calcaneonavicular bar as the associated anomaly. Complete excision of the bar, with interposition of the extensor digitorum brevis muscle, appears a satisfactory method of treatment when done at a sufficiently early age.

Adolescent Bunions

Decision-making in bunion surgery. Mann RA, in Greene WB (ed): American Academy of Orthopaedic Surgeons *Instructional Course Lectures, XXXIX*. Park Ridge, IL, American Academy of Orthopaedic Surgeons, 1990, pp 3-13.

A recognized expert discusses preoperative planning and decision-making in bunion surgery for patients of all ages.

Hallux valgus in the younger patient: The structural abnormality. Houghton GR, Dickson RA. *J Bone Joint Surg* 1979;61B:176-177.

Analysis of 50 patients undergoing osteotomy of the first metatarsal for hallux valgus showed true metatarsus primus varus was not more frequent than in a control series. Intermetatarsal angle was greater in affected feet than in controls. Structural abnormality in hallux valgus is caused by valgus disposition of subsequent metatarsals, rather than varus inclination of the first metatarsal.

Bunions in children: Treatment with a modified Mitchell osteotomy. Luba R, Rosman M. *J Pediatr Orthop* 1984;4:44-47.

Modifications to the original Mitchell osteotomy were made to simplify the surgical technique, improve stability, and facilitate healing and remodeling at the osteotomy site. Long-term results in 45 feet have been excellent.

Surgery for adolescent hallux valgus. Helal B. *Clin Orthop* 1981;157:50-63.
Reviews a number of operations to correct adolescent hallux valgus and factors that influence the outcome. A consistently reliable procedure was the modified Wilson metatarsal shaft osteotomy, which narrows the forefoot, relaxes soft tissues, and maintains excellent mobility of the first metatarsal joint.

Correctional osteotomy for metatarsus primus varus and hallux valgus. Carr CR, Boyd BM. *J Bone Joint Surg* 1968;50A:1353-1367.
Of 90 feet in 51 patients who underwent distal osteotomy of the first metatarsal bone for metatarsus primus varus and hallux varus, results were satisfactory in all but six. Unsatisfactory results were associated with excessive shortening of the first ray or dorsal displacement of the distal fragment.

Dorsal bunions in children. McKay DW. *J Bone Joint Surg* 1983;65A:975-980.
Iatrogenic dorsal bunions in children, observed mostly after operation for post-poliomyelitic paralysis or clubfoot, have been successfully treated surgically by transferring the tendons of the flexor brevis and the abductor and adductor muscles of the hallux to the neck of the first metatarsal. Of 17 feet so treated, only one failure was recorded.

Operative correction of the metatarsus varus primus in hallux valgus. Lapidus PW. *Surg Gynecol Obstet* 1934;58:183-191.
Gives the classic description by Lapidus of his procedure for correction of metatarsus varus primus.

Hallux rigidus. Mann RA, in Greene WB (ed): American Academy of Orthopaedic Surgeons *Instructional Course Lectures, XXXIX*. Park Ridge, IL, American Academy of Orthopaedic Surgeons, 1990, pp 15-21.
The author describes the etiology, clinical history, and typical physical examination findings in hallux rigidus. Different surgical techniques are described. Young people should be considered for chilectomy as previous studies by the author have demonstrated satisfactory pain relief with maintenance of joint function.

The pathogenesis of hallux rigidus. McMaster MJ. *J Bone Joint Surg* 1978;60B:82-87.
In a clinical, radiologic, and pathologic study of hallux rigidus affecting nine toes in seven patients, characteristic chondral and osteochondral lesions, seen to occur at a specific site on the metatarsal head, accounted for the limited dorsiflexion but relatively unrestricted plantarflexion typical of hallux rigidus.

Congenital Short Achilles Tendon

Habitual toe-walkers: A clinical and electromyographic gait analysis. Griffin PP, Wheelhouse WW, Shiavi R, et al. *J Bone Joint Surg* 1977;59A:97-101.
> Electromyographic techniques were used to examine six children who were habitual toe-walkers. Initial gait evaluation showed abnormal muscle synergy patterns during the toe-toe gait and the heel-toe gait. All patients exhibited normal electromyographic patterns after cast treatment.

Congenital short tendo calcaneus. Hall JE, Salter RB, Bhalla Sk. *J Bone Joint Surg* 1967;49B:695-697.
> Toe walking in children who are otherwise normal may be caused by congenital short tendo calcaneus. Tendon lengthening gave good results in 20 patients with this condition.

Hereditary tendo Achillis contractures. Katz MM, Mubarak SJ. *J Pediatr Orthop* 1984;4:711-714.
> Tendo Achillis contracture is a benign condition, but presents cosmetic and functional problems to the patient. This disorder responds well to a short course of casting and follow-up exercises to maintain normal ankle motion and gait. No surgery was necessary for the eight patients in this study.

Osteochondroses of the Foot

Köhler's disease of the tarsal navicular: Long-term follow-up of 12 cases. Ippolito E, Ricciardi Pollini PT, Falez F. *J Pediatr Orthop* 1984;4:416-417.
> Review of 12 patients with Kohler's disease at an average 33-year follow-up found all patients asymptomatic and without radiographic evidence of degenerative change. The type of treatment did not affect time required for bone restoration (average eight months), but did affect duration of pain. Weightbearing plaster cast decreased local pain much faster than a simple arch support.

Köhler's disease of the tarsal navicular. Williams GA, Cowell HR. *Clin Orthop* 1981;158:53-58.
> Long-term results in 20 patients with Köhler's disease of the tarsal navicular suggested that all eventually had spontaneous reconstitution of the navicular and excellent recovery of function.

Osteochondritis dissecans of the talus: Use of the high resolution computed tomography scanner. Zinman C, Reis ND. *Acta Orthop Scand* 1982;53:697-700.
> High resolution computed tomography scanning confirmed the diagnosis (when in doubt) of osteochondritis dissecans of the talus in 12 patients. It also determined the precise location and extent of the lesion, thereby indicating the surgical approach and the area that required drilling. (Ed

note: Recent case reports suggest that magnetic resonance imaging is preferable to computed tomography for this lesion.)

Osteochondral lesions of the talus. Canale St, Belding RH. *J Bone Joint Surg* 1980;62A:97-102.
> Retrospective study of 31 ankles in 29 patients with osteochondral lesions showed that lateral lesions are more likely to cause persistent symptoms than are medial lesions. Necessity for surgery can be determined in part by Berndt and Harty classification, with all stage IV lesions requiring early operation. Degenerative changes were present in 50% of ankle joints regardless of treatment.

Bursitis of the posterior part of the heel: Evaluation of surgical treatment of eighteen patients. Keck SW, Kelly PJ. *J Bone Joint Surg* 1965;47A:267-273.
> When tendo achillis bursitis associated with prominence of the superior part of the tuberosity of the calcaneus does not respond to conservative treatment, it may be necessary to excise the prominence. Good results were obtained in 19 of 26 patients treated by excision or osteotomy. Osteotomy required a longer convalescence.

Köhler's disease of the tarsal scaphoid: An end-result study. Karp MG. *J Bone Joint Surg* 1937;19:84-96.
> This syndrome occurs predominantly in males between 2.5 and 7.5 years of age. Pain, swelling, limping, and localized tenderness in the foot are the most common symptoms. It is more often unilateral than bilateral. Its characteristic radiograph is unrelated to the duration of symptoms or to treatment. Complete regeneration of the bone takes place in an average of 2.75 years, and a normal foot is the usual end result.

Limb-Length Discrepancy

David P. Roye Jr, MD

Modern techniques in limb lengthening: Section I: Symposium. Paley D, (ed). *Clin Orthop* 1990;250:2-159.

> This group of articles includes classics, basic science, several operative techniques and a discussion of complications. The papers are well referenced. This is probably the best single reference on recent developments on this topic.

Assessment and prediction in leg-length discrepancy. Moseley CF. In Barr JS Jr (ed): American Academy of Orthopaedic Surgeons *Instructional Course Lectures, XXXVIII.* Park Ridge, IL, American Academy of Orthopaedic Surgeons, 1989, pp 325-330.

> Describes in detail the straight-line method of predicting leg-length discrepancy.

Skeletal age estimation in leg length discrepancy. Cundy P, Paterson D, Morris L, et al. *J Pediatr Orthop* 1988;8:513-515.

> This article defines the dangers of one-time, bone-age determination in the prediction of leg-length discrepancy.

Pattern of growth retardation after Blount stapling: A Roentgen stereophotogrammetric analysis. Bylander B, Hansson LI, Selvik G. *J Pediatr Orthop* 1983;3:63-72.

> Thirty-one stapled and 25 intact growth regions of distal femur or proximal tibia were studied longitudinally. A uniform pattern of growth retardation was noted after stapling; the retardation was more pronounced and rapid with more advanced skeletal age. Five of 31 had significant asymmetric growth.

Developmental patterns in lower-extremity length discrepancies. Shapiro F. *J Bone Joint Surg* 1982;64A:639-651.

> Five patterns of growth inhibition were noted in patients of the Growth Study Unit established by Green and Anderson. The author believes the straight-line graph of growth inhibition method may lead to inaccurate projections in some of these patterns.

Growth and predictions of growth in the lower extremities. Anderson M, Green WT, Messner MB. *J Bone Joint Surg* 1963;45A:1-14.

> Presents a compilation of yearly growth, evaluated longitudinally, in 100 children (50 boys, 50 girls) from age 8 (girls) or 10 (boys) until cessation of growth. Explains the development of the growth charts and

discusses the value of the skeletal age in older children and the method of using the charts, which are now standard.

Functional Effects

Clinical symptoms and biomechanics of lumbar spine and hip joint in leg length inequality. Friberg O. *Spine* 1983;8:643-651.

> A well-referenced discussion of the biomechanics of leg-length discrepancy precedes a clinical study of Finnish Army conscripts and other patients with chronic hip or back symptoms. Describes a radiographic method for evaluating leg-length discrepancy. Shoe lifts are often recommended.

Lumbar spine structural changes associated with leg length inequality. Giles LG, Taylor JR. *Spine* 1982;7:159-162.

> The authors found concavities of the end plates of lumbar vertebral bodies, wedging of the fifth lumbar vertebra, and traction spurs associated with leg-length inequality of greater than 9 mm in 100 randomly chosen films in a population of non-acute low back pain. No relationship to symptoms is suggested.

Etiology

Leg length discrepancy after femoral shaft fractures in children: Review after skeletal maturity. Stephens MM, Hsu LCS, Leong JCY. *J Bone Joint Surg* 1989;71B:615-618.

> An excellent summary of the literature on leg-length discrepancy secondary to femoral fracture. The fourteen references include most series on this subject.

The influence on the spine of leg-length discrepancy after femoral fracture. Gibson PH, Papaioannou T, Kenwright J. *J Bone Joint Surg* 1983;65B:584-587.

> Fifteen patients with leg-length discrepancy of 1.5 cm or more as a result of femoral fractures sustained between ages 15 and 21 were reviewed at least 10 years after injury. Spines were mobile. No one complained, and neither structural abnormalities nor degenerative changes were seen on radiographs.

Classification and management of congenital abnormalities of the femur. Gillespie R, Torode IP. *J Bone Joint Surg* 1983;65B:557-568.

> Sixty-five patients with more severe varieties of congenitally short femur were classified into two groups. In group I, the hip and knee joints could be made functional and leg equalization was possible in at least some cases. Group II had true proximal femoral focal deficiency, and lengthening was not feasible.

Measurement

Limb-length discrepancy measured with computerized axial tomographic equipment. Huurman WW, Jacobsen FS, Anderson JC, et al. *J Bone Joint Surg* 1987;69A:699-705.
Determines that computerized tomography is more accurate and delivers less radiation than standard orthoroentgenograms in measurement of leg-length discrepancy.

Measurement of leg length inequalities by Micro-Dose digital radiographs. Altongy JF, Harcke HT, Bowen JR. *J Pediatr Orthop* 1987;7:311-316.
Describes validity of a number of digital techniques for measuring leg-length discrepancy.

A straight-line graph for leg-length discrepancies. Moseley CF. *J Bone Joint Surg* 1977;59A:174-179.
This classic article presents in detail the concept and usage of the straight-line graph.

Orthoroentgenography as a method of measuring the bones of the lower extremities. Green WT, Wyatt GM, Anderson M. *J Bone Joint Surg* 1946;28:60-65.
Describes the rationale and technique of orthoroentgenography, sometimes called scanography, and compares this method with teleoroentgenography.

Lengthening

Epiphyseal distraction monitored by strain gauges: Results in seven children. Jones CB, Dewar ME, Aichroth PM, et al. *J Bone Joint Surg* 1989;71B:651-656.
This review of a recent series of patients treated with epiphyseal distraction illustrates some of the difficulties with this technique.

Metaphyseal and physeal lengthening. Price CT. In Barr JS Jr (ed): American Academy of Orthopaedic Surgeons *Instructional Course Lectures, XXXVIII*. Park Ridge, IL, American Academy of Orthopaedic Surgeons, 1989, pp 331-336.
This brief discussion outlines the techniques and indications of distraction osteogenesis and distraction epiphysiolysis.

Current techniques of limb lengthening. Paley D. *J Pediatr Orthop* 1988;8:73-92.
This exhaustive review of current thought in limb lengthening includes an excellent bibliography.

Longitudinal growth of the femur and tibia after diaphyseal lengthening. Shapiro E. *J Bone Joint Surg* 1987;69A:684-690.

Eighteen patients were followed to maturity to assess the effect of subsequent growth on lengthening. Femurs grew faster and tibias slower.

Operative lengthening of the femur. Wagner H. *Clin Orthop* 1978;136:125-142.

Presents a complete discussion of indications, preoperative considerations, operative technique, postoperative care, and results in 58 patients; includes information on problems and complications.

Shortening

Closed shortening of the femur. Blair VP III, Schoenecker PL, Sheridan JJ, et al. *J Bone Joint Surg* 1989;71A:1440-1447.

The technical difficulty of performing closed shortening is emphasized in this review of 20 skeletally mature patients. Results were generally excellent, but complications were reported.

Tibial shortening for leg length discrepancy. Broughton NS, Olney BW, Menelaus MB. *J Bone Joint Surg* 1989;71B:242-245.

Reports long-term follow-up on 12 patients with tibial shortening, an easier alternative to lengthening.

Closed intramedullary osteotomies of the femur. Winquist RA. *Clin Orthop* 1986;212:155-164.

Reviews long-term experience with 154 patients with discrepancies from 2 to 12 cm. Techniques are described and complications discussed.

Epiphysiodesis

Epiphysiodesis: Evaluation of a new technique. Ogilvie JW. *J Pediatr Orthop* 1986;6:147-149.
Percutaneous epiphysiodesis: Experimental study and preliminary clinical results. Canale ST, Russell TA, Holcomb RL. *J Pediatr Orthop* 1986;6:150-156.

These two articles, published together, illustrate the latest approach to epiphysiodesis.

Epiphysiodesis for limb length inequality: Results and indications. Stephens DC, Herrick W, MacEwen GD. *Clin Orthop* 1978;136:41-48.

Presents results of epiphysiodesis in 56 patients with average 10-year follow-up. Discusses patient evaluation and surgical technique.

Epiphysiolysis

Epiphysiolysis for partial growth plate arrest: Results after four years or at maturity. Broughton NS, Dickens DRV, Cole WG, et al. *J Bone Joint Surg* 1989;71B:13-16.
> Reinforces what has been learned about epiphysiolysis in a small group followed to maturity.

Principles of physeal bridge resection. Burke SW. In Barr JS Jr (ed): American Academy of Orthopaedic Surgeons *Instructional Course Lectures, XXXVIII*. Park Ridge, IL, American Academy of Orthopaedic Surgeons, 1989, pp 337-341.
> Briefly outlines techniques for identifying, managing, and predicting the course of physeal bridges.

Congenital Limb Deficiency and the Child Amputee

John A. Herring, MD

Characteristics of the child amputee population. Krebs DE, Fishman S. *J Pediatr Orthop* 1984;4:89-95.
> A review of the characteristics of the patient population of 45 child amputee clinics in the United States and Canada representing a review of 4,105 patients.

The timed appearance of some congenital malformations and orthopaedic abnormalities. Fuller DJ, Duthie RB. In American Academy of Orthopaedic Surgeons *Instructional Course Lectures, XXIII*. St. Louis, CV Mosby, 1974, pp 53-61.
> A review of embryology relevant to congenital malformations that makes it possible to estimate the timing of the insult to the fetus. The article also describes patterns of malformation when multiple abnormalities are present.

Integration of pediatric amputees and their parents with an adult amputee support group. Cammack S. *Assoc Children's Prosthet-Orthot Clin J* 1989;24:6-7.
> This article describes the formation of a support group for amputees that includes both children and adults. The advantages of such a combination include having role models for the children.

A study of stump growth in children with below-knee amputations. Christie J, Lamb DW, McDonald JM, et al. *J Bone Joint Surg* 1979;61B:464-465.
> A review of 20 below-knee amputations, detailing growth of the proximal tibial epiphysis. In limbs amputated for congenital deformity growth was 36% of normal.

Amputation following meningococcemia: A sequela to purpura fulminans. Jacobsen ST, Crawford AH. *Clin Orthop* 1984;185:214-219.
> A review of the pathophysiology and early management of patients with purpura fulminans.

Purpura fulminans: A case for heparin therapy. Chenaille PJ, Horowitz ME. *Clin Pediatr* 1989;28:95-98.
> This brief article from the pediatric literature suggests that heparinization may reverse the coagulopathy associated with purpura fulminans. This, in turn, may somewhat limit tissue destruction and improve amputation level in these patients. The article also describes full compartment

fasciotomies to relieve compartment pressure associated with purpura fulminans.

The major determinants in normal and pathological gait. Saunders JB de CM, Inman VT, Eberhart HD. *J Bone Joint Surg* 1979;61B:464-465.
>This classic article introduces and explains the concepts of the six determinants of gait.

Classification

A classification for congenital limb malformation. Swanson AB, Swanson GD, Tada K. *J Hand Surg* 1983;8:693-702.
>A classification that has been especially used to describe upper-extremity defects.

Dysmelia: A classification and a pattern of malformation in a group of congenital defects of the limbs. Henkel L, Willert H-G. *J Bone Joint Surg* 1969;51B:399-414.
>The authors provide a comprehensive classification system of congenital limb deficiencies based on a review of 287 children. Teratologic sequences are devised that demonstrate the continuous spectra of deformity from least to greatest degree of involvement.

Congenital skeletal limb deficiencies. Frantz CH, O'Rahilly R. *J Bone Joint Surg* 1961;43A:1202-1224.
>A classic article with explanation of the Frantz-O'Rahilly classification of limb deficiencies. Case examples are given to clarify the classification system.

Congenital aplasia and dysplasia of the tibia with intact fibula: Classification and management. Jones D, Barnes J, Lloyd-Roberts GC. *J Bone Joint Surg* 1978;60B:31-39.
>A classic article describing the currently used classification of congenital absence and dysplasia of the tibia.

Congenital Constriction Band Syndrome

Clinical and experimental studies of the congenital constriction band syndrome, with an emphasis on its etiology. Kino Y. *J Bone Joint Surg* 1975;57A:636-643.
>An experimental study in rat fetuses showing that a syndrome resembling constriction band syndrome can be produced by amniocentesis. The deficits were caused, not by constricting bands, but by excessive uterine contraction, which produced hemorrhages in the digits.

Spontaneous intra-uterine amputation. Glessner JR Jr. *J Bone Joint Surg* 1963;45A:351-355.

> Documents the occurrence of intrauterine amputations associated with constricting bands. This type of problem is differentiated from the terminal deficiency type of congenital deficiency.

Congenital constriction band syndrome. Askins G, Ger E. *J Pediatr Orthop* 1988;8:461-466.

> This review of 55 patients with constriction band syndrome gives an overview of the manifestations of this disorder. The occurrence of neurological deficits distal to the constriction bands is documented. Surgical treatment is briefly described.

Proximal Femoral Focal Deficiency

Current concept review: Proximal femoral focal deficiency. Epps CH Jr. *J Bone Joint Surg* 1983;65A:867-870.

> A concise topic review with reference to Aitken's classification and treatment recommendations.

Classification and management of congenital abnormalities of the femur. Gillespie R, Torode IP. *J Bone Joint Surg* 1983;65B:557-568.

> This article reviews 69 patients and divides them into two main groups. The division is made on the basis of long-term surgical and prosthetic management.

Rotationplasty of the lower limb for congenital defects of the femur. *J Bone Joint Surg* 1983;65B:569-573.

> The operative technique for rotation-plasty of the foot (Van Ness) is discussed in detail.

Congenital abnormalities of the femur and related lower extremity malformations: Classification and treatment. Pappas A, *J Pediatr Orthop* 1983;3:45-60.

> New system of classification of proximal femoral focal deficiency is proposed taking into account embryological, teratological, biological, and anatomical considerations of 125 patients with 139 affected femora. Treatment objectives including pelvic-femoral stability, prosthetic management, extremity length equality, knee stability, ankle and foot stability, and anatomical alignment are discussed.

The natural history and early treatment of proximal femoral dysplasia. Fixsen JA, Lloyd-Roberts GC. *J Bone Joint Surg* 1974;56B:86-95.

> Draws attention to the importance of diagnosing those patients who will develop instability due to proximal femoral focal deficiency. Indications for and selection of procedures are discussed for the unstable type.

Proximal femoral focal deficiency: Treatment and classification in 42 cases. Lange DR, Schoenecker PL, Baker CL. *Clin Orthop* 1978;135:15-25.
> Describes the management of proximal focal femoral deficiencies in 42 patients. A new four-part classification introduced is stated to be easier to apply and more useful clinically than the Aitken classification.

Proximal Femoral Focal Deficiency: A Congenital Anomaly. Aitken GT (ed). Washington, DC, National Academy of Sciences, 1969.
> A monograph devoted to proximal focal femoral deficiency. Includes detailed coverage of embryology, classification, natural history, treatment options, and results.

Iliofemoral fusion for proximal femoral focal deficiency. Steel HH, Lin PS, Betz RR, et al. *J Bone Joint Surg* 1987;69A:837-843.
> This article describes a surgical procedure for fusing the femoral condyles to the pelvis, allowing the existing knee joint to act as a hip in a patient with a severe proximal femoral focal deficiency. The author reports four patients, two of whom also had Van Ness rotationplasty, and two of whom had Syme's amputations. The patients with Syme's amputations had a better result that those with the Van Ness. Two patients also required subsequent osteotomy of the femur to improve alignment.

Surgical Management

General

Epiphyseal transplant in amputations: Effects on overgrowth in a rabbit model. Wang GJ, Baugher WH, Stamp WG. *Clin Orthop* 1978;130:285-288.
> Describes a rabbit model in which simple transplantation of epiphyseal units (metatarsal heads) prevented overgrowth of the transected tibia.

Reflections on amputation stumps. Mercer W. (Proceeding: The Ruscoe Clarke Memorial Lecture.) *J Bone Joint Surg* 1963;45B:218-219.
> Emphasizes the importance of surgical technique in producing functional amputation stumps. Emphasizes the importance of myodesis, creation of tibiofibular cross union, and proper management of nerve ends.

Upper-Extremity Surgery

Toe transfers for congenital hand defects. Gilbert A. *J Hand Surg* 1982;7:118-124.
> Describes the technique, indications, and results of microvascular transfer of the second toe to reconstruct congenital hand defects.

The angulation osteotomy of above-elbow stumps. Marquardt E, Neff G. *Clin Orthop* 1974;104:232-238.

Describes an angulation osteotomy of the humerus that improves prosthetic suspension and rotational control in the above-elbow amputee.

The Krukenberg procedure in the juvenile amputee. Swanson AB. *J Bone Joint Surg* 1964;46A:1540-1548.

This classic article describes the technique of the Krukenberg procedure. The four children described had bilateral congenital absence of the hands. The unilateral Krukenberg stump became the dominant useful extremity.

Lower-Extremity Surgery

Disarticulation of the knee in children: A functional assessment. Loder RT, Herring JA. *J Bone Joint Surg* 1987;69A:1155-1160.

This study analyzes the gait and functional abilities after knee disarticulation. Mild gait deviations were documented. The functional level of the children was shown to be satisfactory and better than that reported for above-knee amputation. Prosthetic problems were minimal. The authors conclude that this is a very satisfactory amputation level.

Congenital longitudinal deficiency of the tibia. Schoenecker PL, Capelli AM, Millar EA, et al. *J Bone Joint Surg* 1989;71A:278-287.

A review of 57 patients with variations of tibial deficiency. Describes the results of various means of management including knee disarticulation, Syme's amputation, and the Browne procedure. Recurrent knee flexion contractures routinely occurred after the Browne procedure.

Treatment of hemimelias of the lower extremity: Long-term results. Epps CH Jr, Schneider PL. *J Bone Joint Surg* 1989;71A:273-277.

This paper provides an overview of management of patients with tibial and fibular hemimelia and focuses on early surgical intervention--usually amputation.

The Gruca operation for congenital absence of the fibula. Thomas IH, Williams PF. *J Bone Joint Surg* 1987;69B:587-592.

This article describes a rediscovered procedure in which a tibial osteotomy attempts to create a lateral buttress for the talus. The operation is recommended for children with fibular hemimelia without a great deal of shortening or deformity at birth. The results were satisfactory in 8 of 9 patients.

Syme's amputation: The technical details essential for success. Harris RI. *J Bone Joint Surg* 1956;38B:614-632.

This classic article covers the history and technical details of the Syme amputation.

Congenital absence of the fibula. Coventry MB, Johnson EW Jr. *J Bone Joint Surg* 1952;34A:941-956.
>   This classic article describes the treatment of fibular hemimelia before recognition of the Syme amputation as a more functional procedure.

Congenital longitudinal deficiency of the fibula: Follow-up of treatment by Syme amputation. Westin GW, Sakai DN, Wood WL. *J Bone Joint Surg* 1976;58A:492-496.
>   This study of 42 patients with fibular hemimelia describes the excellent functional results achieved by early Syme amputation.

The Syme amputation in children. Davidson WH, Bohne WH. *J Bone Joint Surg* 1975;57A:905-909.
>   This review of 23 children with Syme amputations describes (1) the suture of extensor tendons to the heel pad, (2) the disarticulation of the ankle without disturbing the distal tibia or fibula, and (3) vascular anomalies, which can involve the posterior tibial artery.

Syme amputation: An evaluation of the physical and psychological function in young patients. Herring JA, Barnhill B, Gaffney C. *J Bone Joint Surg* 1986;68A:573-578.
>   This article reviews the functional activities of patients having a Syme's amputation, most of them for fibular hemimelia. Demonstrates that these children can be expected to participate in normal sports activities, even at a competitive level. There is minimal morbidity or functional loss associated with this amputation level.

Syme's amputation in insensitive feet: A review of twenty cases. Srinivasan H. *J Bone Joint Surg* 1973;55A:558-562.
>   A follow-up study of 20 Syme amputations in patients with insensitive feet due to leprosy. Fifteen patients did well and five had breakdown problems. Heel pad migration was not well tolerated.

Leg-length inequality in children treated by Syme's amputation. Fergusson CM, Morrison JD, Kenwright J. *J Bone Joint Surg* 1987;69B:433-436.
>   This is a review of 37 children who underwent a Syme's amputation for management of leg-length discrepancy with congenital abnormalities of the lower extremity. The results were quite good. The authors recommend Syme's amputation when the predicted leg-length discrepancy is over 15 cm and there are abnormalities of the foot.

The Syme amputation in patients with congenital pseudarthrosis of the tibia. Jacobsen ST, Crawford AH, Millar EA, et al. *J Bone Joint Surg* 1983;65A:533-537.
>   A review of eight patients with congenital pseudarthrosis of the tibia treated with Syme amputation. While the pseudarthrosis did not heal, the patients were functional Syme prosthesis users.

Boyd and Syme ankle amputations in children. Eilert RE, Jayakumar SS. *J Bone Joint Surg* 1976;58A:1138-1141.

> A comparison of Boyd and Syme amputations in children. No distinct advantage was demonstrated for either technique. Details of heel pad management are emphasized.

Partial foot amputations in children: A comparison of the several types with the Syme amputation. Greene WB, Cary JM. *J Bone Joint Surg* 1982;64A:438-443.

> This article evaluates partial foot amputations and compares them with Syme's amputation. Function and prosthetic management were best for transmetatarsal, tarsometatarsal, and midtarsal amputations. A Chopart's level amputation with equinus contracture did not function as well as a Syme's level amputation.

Prosthetic Management

Atlas of Limb Prosthetics: Surgical and Prosthetic Principles. American Academy of Orthopaedic Surgeons. St. Louis, CV Mosby Co, 1981.

> This comprehensive reference source reviews all aspects of prosthetic management of amputees.

Energy cost of walking of amputees: The influence of level of amputation. Waters RL, Perry J, Antonelli D, et al. *J Bone Joint Surg* 1976;58A:42-46.

> A study of energy expenditure during walking, showing that the higher the level of amputation, the greater the energy cost. Patients usually compensate by walking more slowly. When energy demands exceed 50% of maximum aerobic capacity, rapid fatigue will occur.

Prostheses for the child amputee. Sauter WF. *Orthop Clin North Am* 1972;3:483-494.

> A description of the special prosthetic needs of children with bilateral upper-extremity absence, proximal femoral focal deficiency and forequarter amputation.

The acceptance and rejection of prostheses by children with multiple congenital limb deformities. Nichols PJR, Rogers EE, Clark MS, et al. *Artif Limbs* 1968;12:1-13.

> A review of factors involved in acceptance of prostheses, both conventional and powered, by multiply handicapped children. Therapy, psychologic facts, and prosthetic adaptations are discussed in detail.

Management of the child amputee. Aitken GT, Frantz CH. In Reynolds FC (ed): American Academy of Orthopaedic Surgeons *Instructional Course Lectures, XVII*. St. Louis, CV Mosby, 1960, pp 246-295.

> This classic paper covers the whole gamut of management of the child amputee. The article includes much detailed material regarding prosthetic design.

A long-term review of children with congenital and acquired upper-limb deficiency. Scotland TR, Galway HR. *J Bone Joint Surg* 1983;65B:346-349.

> A review of 131 children with upper-extremity limb deficiency shows children most likely to continue using a prosthesis are those with short below-elbow absence who are fitted before age 2. Children with above-elbow amputations and longer below-elbow amputations are unlikely to continue prosthetic use.

Management of severe bilateral upper limb deficiencies. Aitken GT. *Clin Orthop* 1964;37:53-60.

> This classic article details the step-by-step management, from infancy to adolescence, of children with bilateral upper-limb absence.

Age of fitting upper-extremity prostheses in children: A clinical study. MacDonell JA. *J Bone Joint Surg* 1958;40A:655-662.

> This classic article established the rationale for fitting children with upper-extremity prostheses at a very young age.

ISNY flexible sockets for upper-limb amputees. Fishman S, Berger N, Edelstein J. *Assoc Children's Prosthet-Orthot Clin J* 1989;24(1):8-11.

> Flexible thermoplastic sockets are not only more comfortable than rigid sockets, but also allow better heat dissipation and easier adjustments for growth.

Prosthetics in the upper extremity. Lamb DW. *J Hand Surg* 1983;8:774-777.

> This brief overview of developments in upper-extremity prosthetics covers electric and myoelectric design and improved cosmetic approaches.

Management of congenital and acquired amputation in children. Lamb DW, Scott H. Symposium on management of upper-limb amputations. *Orthop Clin North Am* 1981;12:977-994.

> Reviews current developments in conventional and powered prosthetic devices for children with upper-extremity limb deficiencies.

Survey of arm amputees not wearing prostheses: Implications for research and service. Melendez D, LeBlanc M. *Assoc Children's Prosthet-Orthot Clin J* 1988;23(3):62-69.

> This article reviews responses of amputees regarding their prostheses. Problems of appearance and function are evaluated and suggestions made for improving prosthetic practice. The authors feel that many patients are unaware of the options available and that better education will improve prosthetic acceptance.

Comparison of myoelectric and body-powered hands for below-elbow child amputees: 1988 follow-up. Kruger L, Fishman S. *Orthop Trans* 1990, in press.

> This study compared body-powered and myoelectric prostheses in 78 children with a two- to three-year follow-up. Only 44% of study

participants were wearing the myoelectric prosthesis at the study's end, with only 30% using it for active prosthetic prehension--the major purpose for which the device was designed. Advantages of the myoelectric prosthesis were overall appearance, suspension comfort, and a more secure and versatile grasp. Favorable body-powered prosthetic features included lighter weight, coolness, quietness, less inadvertent finger motion, and simplicity of operation. Because pre-school children had limited function from the myoelectric prosthesis, the authors recommend that they be fitted with a different device and that at all ages the myoelectric device be considered in a more critical fashion.

The orthopaedist as prosthetic team leader: Getting the best for your patient from the team. Goldberg B. In Greene WB (ed): American Academy of Orthopaedic Surgeons *Instructional Course Lectures, XXXIX*. Park Ridge, IL, American Academy of Orthopaedic Surgeons, 1990, pp 353-354.
Surgical techniques for conserving tissue and function in lower-limb amputation for trauma, infection, and vascular disease. Bowker JH. In Greene WB (ed): American Academy of Orthopaedic Surgeons *Instructional Course Lectures, XXXIX*. Park Ridge, IL, American Academy of Orthopaedic Surgeons, 1990, pp 355-360.
New concepts in lower-limb amputation and prosthetic management. Pinzur MS. In Greene WB (ed): American Academy of Orthopaedic Surgeons *Instructional Course Lectures, XXXIX*. Park Ridge, IL, American Academy of Orthopaedic Surgeons, 1990, pp 361-366.
Overview of prosthetic feet. Michael JW. In Greene WB (ed): American Academy of Orthopaedic Surgeons *Instructional Course Lectures, XXXIX*. Park Ridge, IL, American Academy of Orthopaedic Surgeons, 1990, pp 367-372.
Current concepts in above-knee socket design. Michael JW. In Greene WB (ed): American Academy of Orthopaedic Surgeons *Instructional Course Lectures, XXXIX*. Park Ridge, IL, American Academy of Orthopaedic Surgeons, 1990, pp 373-378.

> This group of chapters reviews recent advances in lower-extremity amputation and prosthetic management. Although some of the chapters emphasize the dysvascular amputee, the sections on new developments in prosthetic feet and above-knee socket design are particularly germane to the juvenile amputee.

Prosthetic programme after above-knee amputation in children with sarcomata. Cole WG, Klein RW, van Lith M, et al. *J Bone Joint Surg* 1982;64B:586-589.

> The use of an adjustable socket type of temporary prosthesis beginning ten days after amputation for sarcoma is described. Advantages of this simple, early fitting are demonstrated.

Rehabilitation of bilateral lower-extremity amputees. Brown PW. *J Bone Joint Surg* 1970;52A:687-700.

> A classic article devoted to the complexity of overall rehabilitation of bilateral lower-extremity amputees. Four phases of adjustment are described and the psychological aspects of rehabilitation are emphasized.

An innovation in Symes prosthetics. Marx HW. *Orthotics Prosthetics* 1969;23:131-138.

      Describes the fabrication of the double-wall socket with flexible inner shell for a Symes-level prosthesis.

Fractures or Trauma

Richard E. McCarthy, MD
Eric Jones, MD

Fractures in Children. Rockwood CA Jr, Wilkins KE, King RE (eds). Philadelphia, JB Lippincott, 1984, vol 3.
> The most complete and detailed textbook on fractures in the pediatric age group.

Children's Fractures, ed 2. Rang M. Philadelphia, JB Lippincott, 1983.
> The author's unique style, coupled with his vast experience, makes this textbook both educational and enjoyable.

Reaction of the Immature Skeleton to Trauma

The uniqueness of growing bones. Ogden JA. In Rockwood CA Jr, Wilkins KE, King RE (eds): *Fractures in Children.* Philadelphia, JB Lippincott, 1984, vol 3, pp 1-86.
> This reference describes in intricate detail the biomechanical characteristics of growing bones and how they relate to the various fracture patterns seen in the pediatric age group.

The mechanical properties of bone tissue in children. Currey JD, Butler G. *J Bone Joint Surg* 1975;57A:810-814.
> Compares biomechanical properties of long bones in adults and children. Children's bones have a lower modulus of elasticity, a lower bending strength, and lower ash content, and absorb more energy before breaking.

Growth slowdown and arrest lines. Ogden JA. *J Pediatr Orthop* 1984;4:409-415.
> Describes the mechanism for the formation of growth arrest lines that occur after systemic disease or trauma to the extremity.

The anatomy of metaphyseal torus fractures. Light TR, Ogden DA, Ogden JA. *Clin Orthop* 1984;188:103-111.
> Describes the microscopic pattern of torus fractures. Torus fractures occur in the metaphysis because the more porous nature of the cortex allows it to fail in compression.

Plastic deformation in pediatric fractures: Mechanism and treatment. Mabrey JD, Fitch RD. *J Pediatr Orthop* 1989:9:310-314.

The lower mineral content of pediatric bone makes it more plastic than adult bone.

Bone mineral content in children with fractures. Landin L, Nilsson BE. *Clin Orthop* 1983;178:292-296.

Gamma absorptiometry was used to measure bone mineral content in the nonaffected arm of 90 children with fractures. Mineral content was significantly lower in children in whom fractures were caused by low-energy trauma and slightly lower when injuries resulted from high-energy trauma. These findings indicate that endogenous factors may contribute to fractures in children as well as in the elderly.

Injuries to the Physis (Epiphyseal Plate)

Prognosis of epiphysial separation: An experimental study. Dale GG, Harris WR. *J Bone Joint Surg* 1958;40B:116-122.

Experimental studies in monkeys and rabbits demonstrated that healing of physeal injuries occurred by a resumption of the process of endochondral ossification across the fracture site. These types of fractures heal very rapidly.

The vascular contribution to osteogenesis: I. Studies by the injection method. Trueta J, Morgan JD. *J Bone Joint Surg* 1960;42B:97-109.

Injection studies clearly show that the blood vessels that contribute to the growth of the physeal plate originate on the epiphyseal side. The structure and function of the metaphyseal vessels are also defined.

The vascular contribution to osteogenesis: III. Changes in the growth cartilage caused by experimentally induced ischaemia. Trueta J, Amato VP. *J Bone Joint Surg* 1960;42B:571-587.

Demonstrates how ischemia to the epiphyseal vessels causes cessation of growth. Ischemia to the metaphyseal vessels only delays the endochondral ossification process.

Traumatic Separation of the Epiphyses. Poland J. London, Smith, Elder, & Co, 1898.

One of the most complete works ever written on physeal injuries. Still considered a classic. Contains numerous anatomic drawings.

Fractures of the epiphyses. Aitken AP. *Clin Orthop* 1965;41:19-23.

One of the earliest classifications of epiphyseal fractures. Describes three basic types.

Injuries involving the epiphyseal plate. Salter RB, Harris WR. *J Bone Joint Surg* 1963;45A:587-622.

The original classification of physeal injuries into five different types. This is still the most widely accepted classification.

Skeletal Injury in the Child. Ogden JA. Philadelphia, Lea & Febiger, 1982, pp 59-110.
Injury to the growth mechanisms of the immature skeleton. Ogden JA. *Skeletal Radiol* 1981;6:237-253.
> In these two references, Ogden expands the Salter-Harris classification of physeal injuries into nine types with some subgroups.

Surgical treatment of partial closure of the growth plate. Langenskiöld A. *J Pediatr Orthop* 1981;1:3-11.
> Summarizes his original work and includes results of the interposition of fat to reestablish growth of the physis.

Physeal injuries. Bright RW. In Rockwood CA Jr, Wilkins KE, King RE (eds): *Fractures in Children.* Philadelphia, JB Lippincott, 1984, vol 3, pp 87-172.
> Describes in detail the three types of growth arrest patterns. The techniques and indications for surgical repair using silastic elastomer are well illustrated. Summarizes experimental work regarding injuries to the physes.

Physeal injuries of the cervical spine. Lawson JP, Ogden JA, Bucholz RW, et al. *J Pediatr Orthop* 1987;7:428-435.
> This article discusses four cases of injuries to the ring apophysis, two of which were fatal. Discusses the pathomechanics of this injury.

Child-Abuse Syndrome

The battered-child syndrome. Kempe CH, Silverman FN, Steele BF, et al. *JAMA* 1962;181:17-24.
The Battered Child, ed 3. Kempe CH, Helfer RE (eds). Chicago, University of Chicago Press, 1980.
> These two sources discuss the total picture of the child-abuse syndrome and clearly delineate the radiologic manifestations.

The role of orthopedist in child abuse and neglect. Akbarnia BA, Akbarnia NO. *Orthop Clin North Am* 1976;7:733-742.
> Reviews the diagnosis, clinical findings, classification, differential diagnosis, and management of child abuse from an orthopaedic standpoint.

Analysis of 429 fractures in 189 battered children. King J, Diefendorf D, Apthorp J, et al. *J Pediatr Orthop* 1988;8:585-589.
> Of 429 fractures in 189 patients, one half were single fractures, typically occurring in long bones with a transverse pattern. The authors emphasize that a single diaphyseal fracture is more common in battered children than the so-called pathognomonic lesions.

Birth Trauma

The likelihood of injuries when children fall out of bed. Nimityongskul P, Anderson LD. *J Pediatr Orthop* 1987;7:184-186.
> This article reviews 76 children between birth and 16 years of age reported to have fallen out of bed while in the hospital. Severe head, neck, spine, and extemity injuries are extremely rare in children falling out of a hospital bed. If a child is said to have fallen out of bed at home, one should suspect child abuse.

Birth trauma. Gresham EL. *Pediatr Clin North Am* 1975;22:317-328.
> Reviews all types of birth trauma, not just long-bone injuries. Reviews skull and spinal cord injuries as well.

Birth trauma: Incidence and predisposing factors. Levine MG, Holroyde J, Woods JR Jr, et al. *Obstet Gynecol* 1984;63:792-795.
> Reviewed 13,870 live births to find predisposing factors that relate to mechanical birth trauma. A risk assessment profile was developed to identify the fetus at risk. Common injuries were brachial plexus injury, clavicle fracture, and facial nerve injury.

Birth fractures. Bianco AJ, Schlein AP, Kruse RL, et al. *Minn Med* 1972;55:471-474.
> Reviews the types of fractures seen at birth, both those caused by severe trauma and those caused by minimal trauma to abnormal bone. Notes that the initial diagnosis is clinical, because radiographic changes may be delayed.

Neonatal spinal cord injury. Koch BM, Eng GM. *Arch Phys Med Rehabil* 1979;60:378-381.
> Reviews cases of spinal cord injuries that occurred as the result of difficult deliveries. Delineates the clinical picture and notes which levels are compatible with survival.

Brachial plexus birth palsy: A 10-year report on the incidence and prognosis. Greenwald AG, Schute PC, Shiveley JL. *J Pediatr Orthop* 1984;4:689-692.
> Sixty-one cases of brachial plexus birth palsies were documented in 30,451 live births. Prognosis was excellent, with full recovery in 96% of cases. This study shows no decline in the incidence of palsies over 10 years.

Birth fractures in spinal muscular atrophy. Burke SW, Jameson VP, Roberts JM, et al. *J Pediatr Orthop* 1986;6:34-36.
> Presents three patients with birth fractures and Werdnig-Hoffmann disease. Two of the three were erroneously diagnosed as having osteogenesis imperfecta.

Premature Infants

Fractures and rickets in very low birth weight infants: Conservative management and outcome. Koo WWK, Sherman R, Succop P, et al. *J Pediatr Orthop* 1989;9:326-330.
> Seventy-eight infants weighing less than 1,500 grams at birth were followed at periodic intervals until 1 year of age. Approximately one third had evidence of fractures and rickets. Simple splinting was satisfactory management. The rachitic bony changes resolved with increased enteral intake and physical growth.

Fractures in premature infants. Amir J, Katz K, Grunebaum M, et al. *J Pediatr Orthop* 1988;8:41-44.
> Reports fractures occurring in premature infants during the neonatal period. It is postulated that the infants may have bone loss associated with low intake of calcium and phosphorus.

Stress Fractures

On the nature of stress fractures. Stanitski CL, McMaster JH, Scranton PE. *Am J Sports Med* 1978;6:391-396.
> Reviews the recognition and clinical management of stress fractures in young athletes.

Stress fractures in children. Engh CA, Robinson RA, Milgram J. *J Trauma* 1970;10:532-541.
> Describes cases of stress fractures in children under the age of 12 years. Notes that diagnosis can be confused with neoplasms if the child is seen early.

Stress fractures in children. Devas MB. *J Bone Joint Surg* 1963;45B:528-541.
> Reviews the pattern of stress fractures in children. Fibula and tibia are the most common sites. Occasionally these injuries are seen in the pelvis, humerus, and neck of the femur.

Injuries in Children With Generalized Musculoskeletal Diseases

The guarded prognosis of physeal injury in paraplegic children. Wenger DR, Jeffcoat BT, Herring JA. *J Bone Joint Surg* 1980;62A:241-246.
> Notes that physeal injuries were often missed and thus were not immobilized. Of nine cases, five resulted in premature arrest of growth.

Fractures through large non-ossifying fibromas. Drennan DB, Maylahn DJ, Fahey JJ. *Clin Orthop* 1974;103:82-88.

This review of patients with fractures through non-ossifying fibromas recommends biopsy and grafting at the time of fracture, followed by routine immobilization. Immobilization alone failed to heal the lesion.

Pathological fractures in osteomyelitis. Capener N, Pierce KC. *J Bone Joint Surg* 1932;14:501-510.
>One of the earliest descriptions of this complication of chronic osteomyelitis. Recommends prophylactic immobilization to prevent fractures.

Surgical treatment of pathological subtrochanteric fractures due to benign lesions in children and adolescents. Malkawi H, Shannak A, Amr S. *J Pediatr Orthop* 1984;4:63-69.
>Evaluates 12 children and adolescents with pathologic subtrochanteric fractures. Internal fixation allows thorough curettage and bone grafting and results in the least amount of immobilization and the quickest resolution of the lesion and the fracture.

Hand

Fractures of the phalanges of the hand in children. Barton NJ. *Hand* 1979;11:134-143.
>Delineates the fracture patterns of finger fractures seen in a large series in Nottingham, England. While a large percentage of fingertip injuries occur in children, there are very few joint injuries. Physeal fractures are most often Salter-Harris type II.

Rotational supracondylar fractures of the proximal phalanx in children. Dixon GL Jr, Moon NF. *Clin Orthop* 1972;83:151-156.
>Reviews cases of phalangeal neck fractures with 90 degrees of rotation. Very little gross deformity to alert one to the diagnosis. Usually requires surgical intervention.

Management of fractured fingers in the child. Leonard MH, Dubravcik P. *Clin Orthop* 1970;73:160-168.
>Cites experience in 263 phalangeal fractures in children. Of the 263, 75% were treated with simple splintage, 15% required manipulation, and only 10% required surgery (1/3 of these were phalangeal neck fractures). Slightly less than half of the fractures were physeal injuries.

Juxta-epiphysial fracture of the terminal phalanx of the finger. Seymour N. *J Bone Joint Surg* 1966;48B:347-349.
>The mallet finger of childhood is described as a physeal separation rather than avulsion of the tendon. Conservative management and preservation of the nail are emphasized.

Wrist

Fracture of the carpal scaphoid in children: A clinical and roentgenological study of 108 cases. Vahvanen V, Westerlund M. *Acta Orthop Scand* 1980;51:909-913.
> Reviews 108 fractures, most of which were distal. All healed with conservative care. States that classifying the various fracture types in children has no clinical significance.

Non-union of carpal scaphoid fractures in children. Southcott R, Rosman MA. *J Bone Joint Surg* 1977;59B:20-23.
> All eight cases reviewed were treated with bone graft with excellent results.

Injuries of the carpal scaphoid in children. Mussbichler H. *Acta Radiol* 1961;56:361-368.
> Reviews 100 fractures in patients under 15 years of age. Dorsal radial avulsion was seen in 52%. Less than 15% were waist fractures. Emphasizes the need to have views in extreme pronation for full radiographic evaluation. All healed within six weeks.

Forearm

Fractures of the radius and ulna. Evans EM. *J Bone Joint Surg* 1951;33B:548-561.
> Studies 50 cases of forearm fractures treated by conservative methods. Delineates the importance of evaluating (1) the rotational aspects of the fractures, (2) the forces applied at the time of the injury, and (3) the muscles attached to the fragments. Guidelines given regarding rotational position after reduction remain well accepted in the present literature.

Forearm fractures in children: Pitfalls and complications. Davis DR, Green DP. *Clin Orthop* 1976;120:172-183.
> Analyzes 547 forearm fractures and concludes that Evan's rules are not applicable to complete fractures, but can be used for greenstick fractures. Includes statistics regarding complications and incidence of the various fracture patterns.

Pattern of forearm fractures in children. Tredwell SJ, Van Peteghem K, Clough M. *J Pediatr Orthop* 1984;4:604-608.
> Analyzes 500 forearm fractures in children. Noted fracture line tended to progress distally with age. Incidence is three times higher in males. A good article regarding pattern, incidence, and percentages.

The end results of the fractured distal radial epiphysis. Aitken AP. *J Bone Joint Surg* 1935;17:302-308.

Reviews 61 patients with a two- to nine-year follow-up. No residual deformities were seen despite inadequate reduction. Some overgrowth occurs. No osteotomy or repeat manipulation was needed.

Epidemiology of fractures of the distal end of the radius in children as associated with growth. Bailey DA, Wedge JH, McCulloch RG, et al. *J Bone Joint Surg* 1989;71A:1225-1231.

The peak incidence of fractures of the distal end of the radius coincided with the peak velocity of growth in boys and girls. This report did not describe how many of the fractures were physeal injuries versus metaphyseal injuries. Because the peak incidence of fractures could not be explained solely by an increase in physical activity, the authors hypothesize that it may be related to a temporary increase in bone porosity.

Traumatic plastic deformation of the radius and ulna: A closed method of correction of deformity. Sanders WE, Heckman JD. *Clin Orthop* 1984;188:58-67.

Describes the deformities seen with plastic deformation of the radius and/or ulna. Emphasizes that this injury may not be recognized. Describes a unique method of reduction.

Correction with growth following diaphyseal forearm fracture. Högström H, Nilsson BE, Willner S. *Acta Orthop Scand* 1976;47:299-303.
A study of radioulnar movements following fractures of the forearm in children. Daruwalla JS. *Clin Orthop* 1979;139:114-120.
The range of motion following fracture of the shaft of the forearm in children. Nilsson BE, Obrant K. *Acta Orthop Scand* 1977;48:600-602.
Malunited fractures of the forearm in children. Fuller DJ, McCullough CJ. *J Bone Joint Surg* 1982;64B:364-367.
Remodelling after distal forearm fractures in children. (I. The effect of residual angulation on the spatial orientation of the epiphyseal plates; II. The final orientation of the distal and proximal epiphyseal plates of the radius; and III. Correction of residual angulation in fractures of the radius.) Friberg KS. *Acta Orthop Scand* 1979;50:537-546,731-739,741-749.
Remodeling of angulated distal forearm fractures in children. Larsen E, Vittas D, Torp-Pedersen S. *Clin Orthop* 1988;237:190-195.

These six articles analyze forearm fractures and establish guidelines as to which fractures remodel and which have residual angulation or loss of motion. From these six articles one can determine some common prognostic factors in evaluating the adequacy of a reduction.

Cross-union complicating fracture of the forearm: Part II. Children. Vince KG, Miller JE. *J Bone Joint Surg* 1987;69A:654-661.

The authors reviewed ten children who developed cross-union of the radius and ulna following double-bone forearm fractures. No patients had cross-union involving the distal articular part of the forearm. Six cross-unions were in the proximal third of the forearm and were equally distributed between closed and open reduction of the fracture. Four cross-unions developed in the diaphyseal portion of the middle third-distal third and were associated with high-energy injuries. Results after resection seemed to be better in children, but the numbers were too small to allow firm conclusions.

Outpatient treatment of upper extremity injuries in childhood using intravenous regional anaesthesia. Olney BW, Lugg PC, Turner PL, et al. *J Pediatr Orthop* 1988;8:576-579.
> Describes intravenous regional anesthesia in the outpatient department for treatment of 400 upper extremity fractures and dislocations. Anesthesia was safe and effective. Good analgesia was achieved in 90% of the patients. Only nine children (2.3%) had unacceptable reductions requiring further treatment under general anesthesia.

Monteggia Fracture Dislocation

The Monteggia lesion. Bado JL. *Clin Orthop* 1967;50:71-86.
> The classic description and classification of Monteggia injuries into four types. This is the standard classification described in the current literature. This article summarizes the original text published in 1962.

The anterior Monteggia fracture: Observations on etiology and treatment. Tompkins DG. *J Bone Joint Surg* 1971;53A:1109-1114.
> Presents good evidence that type I Monteggia lesions are produced by hyperextension of the elbow, which causes an acute anterior dislocation of the radial head. The total body weight is then transferred to the shaft of the ulna, causing it to fracture. Offers guidelines for treatment based on this mechanism of injury.

Pronation injuries of the forearm: With special reference to the anterior Monteggia fracture. Evans EM. *J Bone Joint Surg* 1949;31B:578-588.
> Evans advocates the hyperpronation theory for type I lesions. His cadaver experiments produced a spiral fracture of the ulna with an associated dislocation of the radial head. He theorized that in a fall on the outstretched arm, the body twisted on a forearm fixed in pronation, creating hyperpronation of the forearm.

The Monteggia fracture with posterior dislocation of the radial head. Penrose JH. *J Bone Joint Surg* 1951;33B:65-73.
> Concludes that type II Monteggia lesions are produced when the elbow is dislocated posteriorly with the forearm supinated.

Greenstick fracture of the upper end of the ulna with dislocation of the radio-humeral joint or displacement of the superior radial epiphysis. Wright PR. *J Bone Joint Surg* 1963;45B:727-731.
> Postulates that type III Monteggia lesions are produced with the elbow extended and the forearm supinated. A varus force applied to the elbow

produces a greenstick fracture of the ulnar metaphysis with a lateral dislocation of the radial head.

The treatment of malunited anterior Monteggia fractures in children. Bell Tawse AJS. *J Bone Joint Surg* 1965;47B:718-723.
Describes the use of a strip of the triceps aponeurosis for reconstructing the orbicular ligament in radial head dislocations that are recognized late.

Monteggia fracture-dislocation in children: Late treatment in two cases. Kalamchi A. *J Bone Joint Surg* 1986;68A:615-619.
Reports two cases of late treatment (3.5 and 6.5 months after injury) for persistent dislocation of the radial head following an unrecognized Monteggia fracture-dislocation. The key to the procedure was osteotomy of the ulna. The radial head could then be relocated and the annular ligament reconstructed.

Elbow

Elbow fat pads with new signs and extended differential diagnosis. Murphy WA, Siegel MJ. *Radiology* 1977;124:659-665.
Expands on displacement of the elbow fat pads in diagnosing intra-articular pathology. Demonstrates how false positive and negative signs can occur.

The normal carrying angle of the elbow: A radiographic study of 422 patients. Beals RK. *Clin Orthop* 1976;119:194-196.
Defines the true carrying angle measurements in males, females, and young children.

Displaced supracondylar fractures of the humerus in children: Treatment by Dunlop's traction. Dodge HS. *J Bone Joint Surg* 1972;54A:1408-1418.
Defines the true measurement of Baumann's angle and how it is affected by various radiographic techniques.

On osteochondrosis deformans juvenilis capituli humeri including investigation of intra-osseous vasculature in distal humerus. Haraldsson S. *Acta Orthop Scand* 1959;38(suppl):1-232.
This monograph reviews in detail the ossification process and vascular supply, both gross and microscopic, of the elbow.

Some vagaries of the capitellum. Silberstein MJ, Brodeur AE, Graviss ER. *J Bone Joint Surg* 1979;61A:244-247.
Some vagaries of the medial epicondyle. Silberstein MJ, Brodeur AE, Graviss ER, et al. *J Bone Joint Surg* 1981;63A:524-528.
Some vagaries of the olecranon. Silberstein MJ, Brodeur AE, Graviss ER, et al. *J Bone Joint Surg* 1981;63A:722-725.
Some vagaries of the lateral epicondyle. Silberstein MJ, Brodeur AE, Graviss ER. *J Bone Joint Surg* 1982;64A:444-448.

Some vagaries of the radial head and neck. Silberstein MJ, Brodeur AE, Graviss ER. *J Bone Joint Surg* 1982;64A:1153-1157.
>This series of five articles describes in detail normal ossification, variations in development, and fracture patterns that may be confused with ossification.

Arthrography in the diagnosis of fractures of the distal end of the humerus in infants. Akbarnia BA, Silberstein MJ, Rende RJ, et al. *J Bone Joint Surg* 1986;68A:599-602.
>Arthrography was used in six infants to clarify the diagnosis of fracture of the distal end of the humerus. The correct diagnosis significantly altered treatment in five of the six.

Supracondylar Humerus Fractures

Experimental hyperextension supracondylar fractures in monkeys. Abraham E, Powers T, Witt P, et al. *Clin Orthop* 1982;171:309-318.
>Describes in detail the pathology involved as to soft-tissue injuries and interposed periosteum. Also describes the positions of stability in maintaining a reduction.

Arterial occlusion in juvenile humeral supracondylar fracture. Rowell PJ. *Injury* 1975;6:254-256.
Dislocation of the brachial artery: A complication of supracondylar fracture of the humerus in childhood. Staples OS. *J Bone Joint Surg* 1965;47A:1525-1532.
>These two articles describe common pathologic findings associated with arterial and/or nerve injuries in supracondylar fractures.

Acute ischemic syndrome: Its treatment; prophylaxis of Volkmann's syndrome. Ottolenghi CE. *Am J Orthop* 1960;2:312-316.
>Delineates common factors responsible for the development of Volkmann's ischemia and defines various types of ischemia, based on the severity of the sequelae.

Transcondylar fractures of the humerus in childhood. Dunlop J. *J Bone Joint Surg* 1939;21:59-73.
>The original article describing the classic Dunlop's skin traction.

Deformity following supracondylar fractures of the humerus. Smith L. *J Bone Joint Surg* 1960;42A:235-252.
Kirschner wire traction in elbow and upper arm injuries. Smith FM. Am J Surg 1947;74:770-787.
Direct skeletal traction in the treatment of fractures. Hey Groves EW. *Br J Surg* 1928;16:149-157.
>The original articles describing the indications and techniques of using olecranon pin traction for treating supracondylar fractures.

Supracondylar fracture of the humerus in children. Palmer EE, Niemann KM, Vesely D, et al. *J Bone Joint Surg* 1978;60A:653-656.
Olecranon screw for skeletal traction of the humerus. Ormandy L. *Am J Surg* 1974;127:615-616.
> These two articles describe the use of a large cancellous screw to apply traction to the olecranon.

Blind pinning of displaced supracondylar fractures of the humerus in children: Sixteen years' experience with long-term follow-up. Flynn JC, Matthews JG, Benoit RL. *J Bone Joint Surg* 1974;56A:263-272.
Percutaneous pin fixation of fractures of the lower end of the humerus. Jones KG. *Clin Orthop* 1967;50:53-69.
Reduction and fixation by pinning "banderillero" style fractures of the humerus at the elbow in children. Casiano E. *Milit Med* 1960;125:262-264.
> These three articles detail the initial use of percutaneous pin fixation for supracondylar fractures. Techniques and pitfalls are described.

Management of displaced extension-type supracondylar fractures of the humerus in children. Pirone AM, Graham HK, Krajbich JI. *J Bone Joint Surg* 1988;70A:641-650 [published erratum appears in *J Bone Joint Surg* 1988;70A:1114].
> In this retrospective study of 230 patients with displaced supracondylar humerus fractures, closed reduction and cast immobilization resulted in a significantly lower percentage of excellent results and a higher percentage of complications. Percutaneous pinning, which provided the highest percentage of excellent results, was advocated as the method of choice for most fractures. However, in cases involving massive soft-tissue swelling or other problems, skeletal traction was acceptable.

Surgical treatment of displaced supracondylar fractures of the humerus in children: Analysis of fifty-two cases followed for five to fifteen years. Weiland AJ, Meyer S, Tolo VT, et al. *J Bone Joint Surg* 1978;60A:657-661.
Open reduction and internal fixation of displaced supracondylar fractures of the humerus in children. Shifrin PG, Gehring HW, Iglesias LJ. *Orthop Clin North Am* 1976;7:573-581.
Immediate open reduction and internal fixation of severely displaced supracondylar fractures of the humerus in children. Ramsey RH, Griz J. *Clin Orthop* 1973;90:130-132.
> These three articles outline the indications, techniques, and pitfalls of open reduction and internal fixation of supracondylar fractures.

Displaced supracondylar fractures of the elbow in children: A report on the fixation of extension and flexion fractures by two lateral percutaneous pins. Fowles JV, Kassab MT. *J Bone Joint Surg* 1974;56B:490-500.
> Describes a large experience with flexion-type supracondylar fractures. Delineates the pathology and principles of treatment. Results were poorer than with extension-type supracondylar fractures.

Supracondylar humeral osteotomy for traumatic childhood cubitus varus deformity. Oppenheim WL, Clader TJ, Smith C, et al. *Clin Orthop* 1984;188:34-39.

> Reviews a large series of osteotomies for cubitus varus. Notes high complication rate (24%) and delineates important technical points to decrease the incidence of complications.

Cubitus varus deformity following supracondylar fractures of the humerus in children. Labelle H, Bunnell WP, Duhaime M, et al. *J Pediatr Orthop* 1982;2:539-546.

> A review of 63 cases of cubitus varus deformity showed no evidence of growth inhibition. The major cause was inadequate reduction with medial tilt. All patients had normal function. Osteotomy to correct the cosmetic effect resulted in 33% unsatisfactory results.

Fractures of the Lateral Condyle

Observations concerning fractures of the lateral humeral condyle in children. Jakob R, Fowles JV, Rang M, et al. *J Bone Joint Surg* 1975;57B:430-436. Injuries of the capitular (lateral humeral condylar) epiphysis. Wadsworth TG. *Clin Orthop* 1972;85:127-142.

> These two articles deal with the types of displacement, treatment, and complications of lateral condyle fractures.

Fractures of the lateral condyle of the humerus in children. Hardacre JA, Nahigian SH, Froimson AI, et al. *J Bone Joint Surg* 1971;53A:1083-1095.

> Details care of 52 patients, including treatment, results, and complications.

Nonunion of slightly displaced fractures of the lateral humeral condyle in children: An update. Flynn JC. *J Pediatr Orthop* 1989;9:691-696.

> The author updates his collected series of this unusual injury. The best treatment for an established nonunion is early stabilization and bone grafting, provided that the fragment is in an acceptable position and that the physis is not closed prematurely.

Non-union of the epiphysis of the lateral condyle of the humerus. Jeffery CC. *J Bone Joint Surg* 1958;40B:396-405.

> Deals with treatment of delayed unions of lateral condyle fractures. Various methods, from screw fixation to simple observation, are advocated.

Fractures of the Medial Condyle

Displaced fractures of the medial humeral condyle in children. Fowles JV, Kassab MT. *J Bone Joint Surg* 1980;62A:1159-1163.

163

Emphasizes that this fracture is often misdiagnosed. A delay in diagnosis or inadequate treatment can cause poor results.

Fracture-separation of the medial humeral condyle in a child confused with fracture of the medial epicondyle. Fahey JJ, O'Brien ET. *J Bone Joint Surg* 1971;53A:1102-1104.
Injury to the lower medial epiphysis of the humerus before development of the ossific center: Report of a case. Cothay PM. *J Bone Joint Surg* 1967;49B:766-767.

These two articles report cases in which fractures of the medial condyle occurred before ossification of the condyle. Each of these was confused with a displaced fracture of the medial epicondyle.

Fractures of the Entire Distal Humeral Physis

Fracture-separation of the distal humeral epiphysis. DeLee JC, Wilkins KE, Rogers LF, et al. *J Bone Joint Surg* 1980;62A:46-51.

Reports a relatively large series of cases. Groups the patients according to age and radiographic appearance and defines principles of treatment. Notes the high incidence of child abuse in infants.

Epiphyseal separation of the distal end of the humerus with medial displacement. Holda ME, Manoli A II, LaMont RI. *J Bone Joint Surg* 1980;62A:52-57.
Fracture-separation of the distal humeral epiphysis in young children. Mizuno K, Hirohata K, Kashiwagi D. *J Bone Joint Surg* 1979;61A:570-573.

These two series (six to seven cases each) describe the risks in treating this injury. Holda's group experienced a high incidence of cubitus varus.

Avascular Necrosis of the Trochlea

Deformity following distal humeral fracture in childhood. Morrissy RT, Wilkins KE. *J Bone Joint Surg* 1984;66A:557-562.

Reports five cases of a rare complication of the distal end of the humerus in children. The deformity produced, the so-called "fishtail" deformity of the distal humerus, may be caused by compromise of the vascular supply to the trochlea.

Fractures of the Medial Epicondyle

Medial epicondyle injuries. Smith FM. *JAMA* 1950;142:396-402.

This classic article reviews a series of 143 cases of epicondylar fracture. Results, which discount many of the previously held concepts regarding these fractures, emphasize that there are very few sequelae and indications for operative intervention.

Fracture of the medial epicondyle with displacement into the elbow joint. Patrick J. *J Bone Joint Surg* 1946;28:143-147.
>Describes the use of Faradic stimulation of the flexor muscles to extract the epicondyle from the joint.

Displacement of the internal epicondyle into the elbow-joint: 4 cases successfully treated by manipulation. Roberts NW. *Lancet* 1934;2:78-79.
>Describes a simple manipulative technique for extracting the medial epicondyle from the joint.

Fractures of the medial epicondyle of the humerus. Bernstein SM, King JD, Sanderson RA. *Contemp Orthop* 1981;637-641.
>This large series of epicondylar fractures emphasizes good results with conservative measures.

Biomechanics of elbow instability: The role of the medial collateral ligament. Schwab GH, Bennett JB, Woods GW, et al. *Clin Orthop* 1980;146:42-52.
Elbow instability and medial epicondyle fractures. Woods GW, Tullos HS. *Am J Sports Med* 1977;5:23-30.
>These two articles define the true function of the various portions of the medial collateral ligament. The valgus stress test to determine elbow stability after a fracture of the medial condyle is described.

Fractures of the Olecranon

A proximal radial metaphyseal fracture presenting as wrist pain. Anderson TE, Breed AL. *Orthopedics* 1982;5:425-428.
>Points out the pitfall of referred pain of radial head fractures to the wrist. Can be a source of an overlooked diagnosis.

Radial head and neck fractures in children. Steinberg EL, Golomb D, Salama R, et al. *J Pediatr Orthop* 1988;8:35-40.
>Analyzes 42 fractures of the neck of the radius in children. Complications were frequent. The authors advocate immobilization for angulation less than 30 degrees, closed manipulation or percutaneous leverage for moderate angulation, and open reduction for angulation greater than 60 degrees.

Displaced radial neck fractures in children. Newman JH. *Injury* 1977;9:114-121.
>Reports a series of 47 injuries. Divides them into five types. Describes radial neck fractures as occurring when an elbow dislocation is reduced. Includes a good review of the complications.

Displaced fractures of the neck of the radius in children. Jones ERL, Esah M. *J Bone Joint Surg* 1971;53B:429-439.

Reviews the various mechanisms of injury. Divides mechanisms into valgus stress and those occurring with elbow dislocations. Outlines some good principles of treatment.

Treatment of displaced transverse fractures of the neck of the radius in children. Patterson RF. *J Bone Joint Surg* 1934;16:695-698.
Outlines the displacement forces that occur with fracture of the radial neck. Describes a manipulative technique.

Fractures of the olecranon in children. Matthews JG. *Injury* 1980;12:207-212.
This extensive review of olecranon fractures in children points out that many of these are part of a complex injury to the joint. Groups the injuries and defines the associated complications.

Elbow Dislocation (Including Isolated Radial Head)

Congenital radial head dislocation. Mardam-Bey T, Ger E. *J Hand Surg* 1979;4:316-320.
Describes features of a congenital dislocation of the radial head that enable the physician to differentiate these radiographic findings from those seen in an acute dislocation.

Entrapment of the median nerve after dislocation of the elbow: A case report. Hallett J. *J Bone Joint Surg* 1981;63B:408-412.
Describes in detail the pathologic findings of an entrapped median nerve after reduction of a dislocated elbow. Defines three types of entrapment patterns.

A radiological sign of entrapment of the median nerve in the elbow joint after posterior dislocation: A report of two cases. Matev I. *J Bone Joint Surg* 1976;58B:353-355.
Describes a grooving in the posterior medial aspect of the distal humerus from pressure on the bone by the entrapped median nerve.

Arterial injury: A complication of posterior elbow dislocation. Louis DS, Ricciardi JE, Spengler DM. *J Bone Joint Surg* 1974;56A:1631-1636.
Demonstrates the anatomic basis for compromise of the collateral circulation when the brachial artery is ruptured secondary to an elbow dislocation. Emphasizes the need for primary repair of the artery.

Anatomic investigations of the mechanism of injury and pathologic anatomy of "pulled elbow" in young children. Salter RB, Zaltz C. *Clin Orthop* 1971;77:134-143.
A thorough and complete discussion of various theories and pathoanatomy concerning the so-called "pulled elbow" in young children.

Recurrent dislocation of the elbow. Osborne G, Cotterill P. *J Bone Joint Surg* 1966;48B:340-346.
> Describes this defect as a failure of reattachment of the posterior lateral aspect of the capsule to the lateral condyle. Delineates a soft-tissue repair technique.

Little League Elbow

Little League survey: The Houston Study. Gugenheim JJ Jr, Stanley RF, Woods GW, et al. *Am J Sports Med* 1976;4:189-200.
Little League survey: The Eugene study. Larson RL, Singer KM, Bergstrom R, et al. *Am J Sports Med* 1976;4:201-209.
> These articles detail the long-term effects of throwing in young individuals. Demonstrates that long-term effects are minimal when moderation is practiced in games.

Injury to the throwing arm: A study of traumatic changes in the elbow joints of boy baseball players. Adams JE. *Calif Med* 1965;102:127-132.
> First to warn of the detrimental effects of excessive throwing by Little League pitchers.

Little leaguer's elbow. Brogdon BG, Crow NE. *Am J Roentgenol* 1960;83:671-675.
> The original radiographic description of medial epicondyle abnormalities associated with excessive throwing in Little League pitchers.

Fractures of the Proximal Humeral Physis

Dislocation of the proximal epiphysis of the humerus in newborns: Report of two cases and discussion of diagnostic criteria. Lemperg R, Liliequist B. *Acta Paediatr Scand* 1970;59:377-380.
> Reports two cases in neonates. Describes the clinical and radiographic picture of this unusual injury, which is differentiated from a pure brachial plexus injury.

Fracture and fracture separation of the proximal humerus in children: Report of 136 cases. Kohler R, Trillaud JM. *J Pediatr Orthop* 1983;3:326-332.
> Reports a large series from France. While 25% were treated surgically, the authors still emphasize the superiority of nonsurgical methods. Believed the hanging arm cast was ineffective.

Fractures involving the proximal humeral epiphyseal plate. Dameron TB Jr, Reibel DB. *J Bone Joint Surg* 1969;51A:289-297.
> Follow-up of 69 patients with displaced fracture of the proximal humeral physis. Emphasizes the good results obtained with closed methods.

Fractures of the proximal humeral epiphysial plate. Neer CS II, Horwitz BS. *Clin Orthop* 1965;41:24-31.

> This classic article reviews long-term results of 89 fractures of the proximal humeral physis. Irreducible fractures often have interposition of the long head of the biceps.

Fracture of the upper end of the humerus in children: A follow-up of 44 cases. Nilsson S, Svartholm F. *Acta Chir Scand* 1965;130:433-439.

> Results of follow up in 44 cases. Those with surgical intervention had poorer results despite a good radiologic appearance.

Little league shoulder. Cahill BR, Tullos HS, Fain RH. *J Sports Med* 1974;2:150-153.

> Describes a chronic stress fracture of the proximal humeral physis in the Little League pitcher.

Clavicle Fractures

Fracture of the outer clavicle in children and adults, abstract. Rockwood CA Jr. *J Bone Joint Surg* 1982;64B:642.

> A brief report detailing the intact periosteum attached to the intact coracoclavicular ligaments in fracture dislocations of the distal clavicle. Recommends conservative measures up to age 16.

Dislocations of the sternoclavicular joint. Rockwood CA Jr. In American Academy of Orthopaedic Surgeons *Instructional Course Lectures, XXIV*. St. Louis, CV Mosby, 1975, pp 144-159.

> Describes the pathology of separation of the physis of the medial end of the clavicle. Up to age 25 these will remodel and need only conservative care.

Acromioclavicular lesions in children. Eidman DK, Siff SJ, Tullos HS. *Am J Sports Med* 1981;9:150-154.

> Reviews acromioclavicular joint lesions in children and adolescents and advocates conservative treatment for patients less than 13 years of age. Describes a lesion in which the failure occurred through the physis of the coracoid process.

Shoulder Dislocations (Glenohumeral Joint)

Fractures and dislocations of the shoulder: Part III. Fractures and dislocations of the ends of the clavicle, scapula, and glenohumeral joint. Rockwood CA Jr. In Rockwood CA Jr, Wilkins KE, King RE (eds): *Fractures in Children.* Philadelphia, JB Lippincott, 1984, vol 3, pp 624-682.

> Classifies dislocations of the glenohumeral joint in children into two major types, traumatic and atraumatic. Gives good guidelines for the

management of each type. Emphasizes that traumatic dislocation before the age of 12 is extremely rare.

Adolescent traumatic dislocations of the shoulder with open epiphyses. Wagner KT Jr, Lyne ED. *J Pediatr Orthop* 1983;3:61-62.
> Reports nine cases of glenohumeral dislocation in patients 12 years of age or older with open epiphyses. Recurrence rate was 80%.

Voluntary dislocation of the shoulder: A preliminary report on a clinical, electromyographic, and psychiatric study of twenty-six patients. Rowe CR, Pierce DS, Clark JG. *J Bone Joint Surg* 1973;55A:445-460.
> A review of 26 patients with voluntary dislocations found that most did well with muscle rehabilitation alone. Advised extreme caution in patients with psychological problems. A combination of procedures, rather than a single procedure, was usually needed for surgical repair.

Fractures of the Spine (Spinal Cord Injuries)

Emergency transport and positioning of young children who have an injury of the cervical spine. Herzenberg JE, Hensinger RN, Dedrick DK, et al. *J Bone Joint Surg* 1989;71A:15-22.
> The cervical spine of children less than 7 years of age is positioned in flexion when they are transported on a standard flat back board. Because of the relatively large circumference of the head in young children, the transport board must have either a recess for the occiput or some other adaptation to prevent undesirable cervical flexion during emergency transport.

Fractures of the odontoid process in young children. Sherk HH, Nicholson JT, Chung SM. *J Bone Joint Surg* 1978;60A:921-924.
Fracture of odontoid process in children. Griffiths SC. *J Pediatr Surg* 1972;7:680-683.
> Reports a series of odontoid fractures in children, all of which were treated by simple immobilization.

Spinal cord injury without osseous spine fracture. Yngve DA, Harris WP, Herndon WA, et al. *J Pediatr Orthop* 1988;8:153-159.
> Patients who developed spinal cord injury without bone injury and children who developed spinal cord injury with an associated spine fracture were compared. The group without bony injury were considerably younger and had injury clustered at the cervicothoracic junction. Extravasation of myelographic dye from the spinal canal was a poor prognostic sign.

Paralytic spinal deformity following traumatic spinal-cord injury in children and adolescents. Lancourt JE, Dickson JH, Carter RE. *J Bone Joint Surg* 1981;63A:47-53.

Deals with the types of spinal deformities that develop with traumatic etiologies in paraplegic children. Updates principles of treatment.

Posterior lumbar apophyseal fractures. Handel SF, Twiford TW Jr, Reigel DH, et al. *Radiology* 1979;130:629-633.
Delineates the vertebral body apophyseal avulsions that often accompany lumbar disk herniation in children and adolescents.

Spinal lesions in battered babies. Cullen JC. *J Bone Joint Surg* 1975;57B:364-366.
Case reports delineating this often-missed injury in abused children. Some cases showed considerable injury to the spine with minimal displacement.

Pelvic Fractures

Growth and development of the acetabulum in the normal child: Anatomical, histological, and roentgenographic studies. Ponseti IV. *J Bone Joint Surg* 1978;60A:575-585.
A detailed description of the growth process of the acetabular cartilage. Essential knowledge for evaluating the effect of pelvic fractures in children.

Treatment of avulsion of the ischial tuberosity. Martin TA, Pipkin G. *Clin Orthop* 1957;10:108-118.
Classifies injuries into three groups: (1) Apophysiolysis: treat conservatively, (2) Acute avulsion fracture: treat with closed or open reduction, (3) Old ununited fracture: treat with excision or repair of hamstring origin. Authors found that many of their cases in group 2 or 3 were symptomatic. Excellent references.

Ischial apophysiolysis: A new syndrome. Milch H. *Clin Orthop* 1953;2:184-193.
This early description has an extensive review of previous case reports dealing with ischial apophysis avulsions. Recommends conservative care. A classic article.

Avulsion injuries of the pelvis and proximal femur. Fernbach SK, Wilkinson RH. *AJR* 1981;137:581-584.
Epiphyseal injuries about the hip joint. Hamsa WR. *Clin Orthop* 1957;10:119-124.
These two articles review the anatomy, incidence, radiographic signs, and clinical findings of the various apophyseal avulsions that occur around the hip joint. Both articles recommend conservative management.

Pelvic disruptions in children. McDonald GA. *Clin Orthop* 1980;151:130-134.

Demonstrates that pelvic fractures in children can result in growth disturbances with pelvic obliquity and leg-length discrepancy.

Pelvic fractures in children: Review of 120 patients with a new look at general management. Reichard SA, Helikson MA, Shorter N, et al. *J Pediatr Surg* 1980;15:727-734.
Fractures of the pelvis and associated injuries in children. Quinby WC Jr. *J Pediatr Surg* 1966;1:353-364.

These articles review internal injuries associated with pelvic fractures. Quinby noted that major disruptions of the sacroiliac joint were accompanied by severe injury to the primary iliac vessels and sciatic nerve. Reichard used balloon catheters to control hemorrhage.

Pediatric pelvic fractures: Review of 52 patients. Bryan WJ, Tullos HS. *J Trauma* 1979;19:799-805.
Pelvic fractures in children. Reed MH. *J Can Assoc Radiol* 1976;27:255-261.

Two large series of pelvic fractures in children, usually as a result of severe trauma. Overall incidence of pelvic fractures was much less than in adults. Most were stable. Acetabular fractures are rarely isolated.

Dislocation of the Hip

Traumatic dislocation of the hip in adolescence with separation of the capital epiphysis: Two case reports. Fiddian NJ, Grace DL. *J Bone Joint Surg* 1983;65B:148-149.
Dislocation of the hip with traumatic separation of the capital femoral epiphysis: Report of a case with successful outcome. Mass DP, Spiegel PG, Laros GS. *Clin Orthop* 1980;146:184-187.

Mass and associates had a good result in their case, which was a younger child. In the other case, the patient was older and the outcome was poor. Good review of this specific injury.

Traumatic anterior dislocation of the hip in childhood. Barquet A. *Injury* 1982;13:435-440.

Reviews data from 111 cases of anterior dislocation reported in world literature. Ratio of anterior to posterior is the same in children as in adults. Allis method most successful in reduction. High incidence of associated injuries.

Natural history of avascular necrosis following traumatic hip dislocation in childhood: A review of 45 cases. Barquet A. *Acta Orthop Scand* 1982;53:815-820.

Reviews outcome of 145 cases followed to maturity. Defines two groups. Younger children's results were similar to Legg-Perthes. In children older than 12, the course was similar to avascular necrosis in the adult. Incidence of deformities was high.

Traumatic dislocation of the hip in children. Offierski CM. *J Bone Joint Surg* 1981;63B:194-197.

Traumatic dislocations and fracture-dislocations of the hip in children. Canale ST. In Salvati EA (ed): *The Hip: Proceedings of the Ninth Open Scientific Meeting of the Hip Society*, 1981. St. Louis. CV Mosby, 1981, pp 219-245.

Traumatic dislocation of the hip in children: Factors influencing prognosis and treatment. Funk FJ Jr. *J Bone Joint Surg* 1962;44A:1135-1145.

> Three major series of traumatic hip dislocations. Canale demonstrated poorer results if there were associated fractures. The epidemiological data are all fairly similar.

Recurrent traumatic dislocation of the hip in childhood. Barquet A. *J Trauma* 1980;20:1003-1006.

> Reviews the world literature on this entity. Recommends surgery only if arthrogram shows an evagination through soft-tissue defect. Believes many spontaneously improve with age as capsule tightens. No factors were found that favored recurrence.

Traumatic dislocation of the hip joint in children: Final report. The Scientific Research Committee of the Pennsylvania Orthopaedic Society. *J Bone Joint Surg* 1968;50A:79-88.

> Describes outcome of 51 cases from Pennsylvania Orthopaedic Society plus nine other series--a total of 165 cases. Defines incidence of avascular necrosis, final outcome and how dislocations differ in children and in adults. An analysis of the data from this article is updated in a later article by Gartland and Benner (*Orthop Clin North Am* 1976;7:687-700).

Fractures of the Femoral Neck and Peritrochanteric Region

Obstetrical fracture-separation of the upper femoral epiphysis. Theodorou SD, Ierodiaconou MN, Mitsou A. *Acta Orthop Scand* 1982;53:239-243.

> Reports five cases with five-year follow-up. An extensive review of the literature. Noted high incidence of breech deliveries. Did not experience varus as previously described. No cases of avascular necrosis.

Stress fracture of the femoral neck in a patient with open capital femoral epiphyses. Wolfgang GL. *J Bone Joint Surg* 1977;59A:680-681.

> Reviews world literature on stress fractures of femoral neck. Relates that most are in young male adults. Describes a case in a ten-year-old female.

Traumatic separation of the upper femoral epiphysis in young children. Ratliff AHC. *J Bone Joint Surg* 1968;50B:757-770.

> Describes 13 cases of strictly transphyseal injuries. Very high complication rate with resultant deformities (11 of 13). Differentiates this from slipped epiphysis.

Fractures of the neck of the femur in children. Ratliff AHC. In Salvati EA (ed): *The Hip: Proceedings of the Ninth Open Scientific Meeting of the Hip Society*, 1981. St. Louis, CV Mosby, 1981, pp 188-218.
> An extensive review of 168 cases. Discusses incidence, types, complication rates, and treatment principles. Supersedes an earlier review of 71 patients (*J Bone Joint Surg* 1962;44B:528-542). Elaborates on his classification of avascular necrosis.

Fracture of the neck and intertrochanteric region of the femur in children. Canale ST, Bourland WL. *J Bone Joint Surg* 1977;59A:431-443.
Fractures of the hip in children from birth to adolescence. Miller WE. *Clin Orthop* 1973;92:155-188.
Fractures of the neck of the femur in children. Lam SF. *J Bone Joint Surg* 1971;53A:1165-1179.
Fractures of the hip in children: Treatment and results. Ingram AJ, Bachynski B. *J Bone Joint Surg* 1953;35A:867-887.
> These four articles include 175 patients. These and Ratliff's series are the ones most quoted in the literature. All use the Delbert-Colonna classification. Incidence of various types of fractures and complication rates are well outlined.

Hip fractures in children. Morrissy R. *Clin Orthop* 1980;152:202-210.
> This excellent review article compares various methods of treatment advocated in the larger published series and compares the overall results.

Fractures of the Femoral Shaft

Lower-extremity balanced traction: A modification of Russell traction. Litchman HM, Duffy J. *Clin Orthop* 1969;66:144-147.
> Delineates the forces acting on the lower extremity with Russell's traction and reemphasizes the proper position of the slings and weights.

Modified Bryant's traction. Ferry AM, Edgar MS Jr. *J Bone Joint Surg* 1966;48A:533-536.
> Demonstrates a modification using a separate knee sling, as with Russell's traction, to decrease the dangerous forces and pressures that occur with Bryant's traction.

The management of complications of femoral shaft fractures in children. Lansche WE, Mishkin MR, Stamp WG. *Southern Med J* 1963;56:1001-1012.
> Delineates the complications associated with open reduction and Bryant's traction in the treatment of femoral shaft fractures in children.

Bryant's traction: A provocative cause of circulatory complications. Nicholson JT, Foster RM, Heath RD. *JAMA* 1955;157:415-418.
> Reports cases with significant sequelae from Bryant's traction. Demonstrated ischemia caused by elevation of the legs and hyperextension of the knee.

Rotational deformities after femoral shaft fractures in childhood: A retrospective study 27-32 years after the accident. Brouwer KJ, Molenaar JC, van Linge B. *Acta Orthop Scand* 1981;52:81-89.

> Long-term follow-up of femoral shaft fractures (27 to 32 years) revealed no significant rotational malalignment using Bryant's and Russell's traction. Felt there was some spontaneous correction of rotational deformities.

The hazards of tibial pin replacement in 90-90 skeletal traction. Miller PR, Welch MC. *Clin Orthop* 1978;135:97-100.

> Demonstrated a high incidence of knee displacement problems (70%) with subsequent disability following 90-90 traction with tibial pins. One case of closure of anterior portion of the proximal tibial physis also occurred.

Skeletal traction for fractures of the femoral shaft in children: A long-term study. Aronson DD, Singer RM, Higgins RF. *J Bone Joint Surg* 1987;69A:1435-1439.

> Fifty-four children treated by 90-90 skeletal traction for fracture of the femur were evaluated. Limb-length discrepancy was more common in children who were 11 years of age or older. These children should be reduced without allowing overriding. Traction pins placed obliquely had a significant association of knee alignment abnormalities.

Displaced fractures of the femoral diaphysis in children: Definitive treatment in a double spica cast. Allen BL Jr, Kant AP, Emery FE. *J Trauma* 1977;17:8-19. Long-term results in the treatment of femoral-shaft fractures in young children by immediate spica immobilization. Irani RN, Nicholson JT, Chung SM. *J Bone Joint Surg* 1976;58A:945-951.

> These articles describe the techniques and merits of immediate spica casts for femoral shaft fractures in infants and children. Indications, acceptable amount of overriding, and angulation are well delineated.

Acute osteomyelitis following closed fractures: Report of three cases. Canale ST, Puhl J, Watson FM, et al. *J Bone Joint Surg* 1975;57A:415-418.

> Delineates the clues to this rare complication of closed femoral shaft fractures. Late onset of pain, unrelieved by immobilization, and local systemic signs of inflammation should be investigated thoroughly.

Remodelling after femoral shaft fracture in children. Viljanto J, Kiviluoto H, Paananen M. *Acta Chir Scand* 1975;141:360-365.

> One of the few articles that follows and quantitates angular malalignment. The greater the angle, the greater the remodeling. Varus remodels 40%, valgus 60%, and ante or recurvatum 70%. Remodeling continued for up to 5 years.

Fractures of the femoral shaft in children: The overgrowth phenomenon. Shapiro F. *Acta Orthop Scand* 1981;52:649-655.

Reviewed 74 patients until maturity. Femoral overgrowth averaged 0.9 cm, with 0.3 cm in tibia. Overgrowth was independent of age, level of fracture, or position of fracture. Overgrowth can continue for 3.5 years following fracture.

Cast brace management of the femoral shaft fracture in children and young adults. Gross RH, Davidson R, Sullivan JA, et al. *J Pediatr Orthop* 1983;3:572-582.
  Delineates a method of early ambulation combined with traction using a femoral pin incorporated into a cast brace. Results were comparable to those seen when traction and casting are used alone.

Management of femoral shaft fractures in the adolescent. Herndon WA, Mahnken RF, Yngve DA, et al. *J Pediatr Orthop* 1989;9:29-32.
  Intramedullary nailing was superior to closed treatment of femur fractures in teenage children (age range 11 to 16 years). Premature growth arrest was not noted in the surgical group.

Femoral intramedullary nailing in the growing child. Ziv I, Blackburn N, Rang M. *J Trauma* 1984;24:432-434.
  A good article delineating the use of intramedullary rods (Rush rods or Kuntscher nails) in young children where other types of management were not successful. Trochanteric epiphyseodesis occurred with K nails. Procedure is effective and safe where indicated.

Treatment of femoral fracture in the child with head injury. Ziv I, Rang M. *J Bone Joint Surg* 1983;65B:276-278.
  Results with intramedullary fixation were better than with traction in spastic, head-injured children. Plate fixation had a high rate of complication. Overgrowth was not a problem. No need to shorten femur at surgery.

Physeal arrest about the knee associated with non-physeal fractures in the lower extremity. Hresko MT, Kasser JR. *J Bone Joint Surg* 1989;71A:698-703.
  The authors describe seven patients who developed physeal arrest of the distal femur or proximal tibia associated with fractures elsewhere in the lower extremity not involving the growth plate. Recognition of growth disturbance was delayed an average of 0.8 years. This article provides another reason why children with long-bone fractures should be followed beyond the time of initial bony healing.

Fractures Involving the Distal Femoral Physis

Growth disturbances following distal femoral physeal fracture-separations. Riseborough EJ, Barrett IR, Shapiro F. *J Bone Joint Surg* 1983;65A:885-893. Fractures of the distal femoral epiphyses: Factors influencing prognosis. A review of thirty-four cases. Lombardo SJ, Harvey JP Jr. *J Bone Joint Surg* 1977;59A:742-751.

These two articles, reviewing 100 cases, demonstrate a high incidence of growth problems in this injury. Juveniles (2 to 11 years) usually sustained highest growth-arrest rate (83%) and also had the most violent injuries. Prognosis is related more closely to the amount of displacement than to the Salter-Harris classification.

Fractures of the Intercondylar Eminence of the Tibia

Fractures and dislocations of the knee. Roberts JM. In Rockwood CA Jr, Wilkins KE, King RE (eds): *Fractures in Children*. Philadelphia, JB Lippincott, 1984, vol 3, pp 891-982.
> Enlarges on his original report, fractures of the condyles of the tibia, in *J Bone Joint Surg* 1968;50A:842. Describes anatomic factors that facilitate closed reduction. Advocates closed reduction in almost all cases.

Fracture of the intercondylar eminence of the tibia. Meyers MH, McKeever FM. *J Bone Joint Surg* 1970;52A:1677-1684.
> This classic article describes a classification based on the degree of displacement. Recommends open reduction and internal fixation in cases with wide displacement.

Fractures Involving the Proximal Tibial Physis

Fractures of the proximal tibial epiphysis. Burkhart SS, Peterson HA. *J Bone Joint Surg* 1979;61A:996-1002.
> Reports 28 cases. Type IV Salter-Harris fractures most often result from lawnmower injuries. Most type I and II injuries occurred in the adolescent age group. Recommends stress films if diagnosis is in doubt. Type III injuries are often associated with avulsion of tibial tubercle.

Fractures of the tibia through the proximal tibial epiphyseal cartilage. Shelton WR, Canale ST. *J Bone Joint Surg* 1979;61A:167-173.
> Reports 39 cases, including two cases of popliteal artery disruption. Other complications included compartment syndrome, peroneal nerve palsy, and associated ligamentous injuries. Age range and fracture patterns were similar to those in Burkhart and Peterson's series (above).

Fractures of the Tibial Tuberosity (Tubercle)

Tibial tuberosity avulsion fracture in adolescents. Christie MJ, Dvonch VM. *J Pediatr Orthop* 1981;1:391-394.
Fracture of the tibial tubercle. Levi JH, Coleman CR. *Am J Sports Med* 1976;4:254-263.

Avulsion fractures of the tibial tubercle. Hand WL, Hand CR, Dunn AW. *J Bone Joint Surg* 1971;53A:1579-1583.

> Three series totaling 30 cases. All were associated with some type of jumping activity. Many had preceding Osgood Schlatter's disease. All were seen at the termination of skeletal maturity. No complications seen with open reduction.

Fractures of the tibial tuberosity in adolescents. Ogden JA, Tross RB, Murphy MJ. *J Bone Joint Surg* 1980;62A:205-215.

> An extensive review of the development of the secondary ossification centers of the tibial tuberosity as they relate to this injury and Osgood Schlatter's Disease. Modifies Watson Jones original classification. Reviews 15 cases with relatively few complications.

Fractures of the Tibial Shaft and Metaphyses

Acquired valgus deformity of the tibia in children. Balthazar DA, Pappas AM. *J Pediatr Orthop* 1984;4:538-541.

> Offers a complete review of the development of this deformity, which can be due either to overgrowth, incomplete reduction, or both. Warns against osteotomy because of recurrent deformity.

Fibrous interposition causing valgus deformity after fracture of the upper tibial metaphysis in children. Weber BG. *J Bone Joint Surg* 1977;59B:290-292.

> Reports some cases explored surgically in which interposed pes anserinus was found. Speculates that this prevented complete reduction, with the result that a deformity developed.

Genu valgum as a complication of proximal tibial metaphyseal fractures in children. Jackson DW, Cozen L. *J Bone Joint Surg* 1971;53A:1571-1578.

> A follow-up on Cozen's original report of this complication of undisplaced tibial metaphyseal fractures. Noted progressive deformity even after immobilization.

Fractures of the tibia in children. Hansen BA, Greiff J, Bergmann F. *Acta Orthop Scand* 1976;47:448-453.

> Longitudinal studies in 102 children. Good article for statistics regarding incidence, age group, time of healing. Found angulation corrected only by 10%, ceased at 18 months, and was independent of age at time of fracture.

Stress fractures in children. Engh CA, Robinson RA, Migram J. *J Trauma* 1970;10:532-541.

> Reported nine cases of stress fractures of the tibia, which were initially misdiagnosed as other entities. An excellent description of the pathologic changes.

Obscure tibial fracture of infants: The toddler's fracture. Dunbar JS, Owen HF, Nogrady MB, et al. *J Can Assoc Radiol* 1964;15:136-144.

> The original description of this fracture, which occurs with minimal clinical and radiographic signs and is often missed initially on routine radiographs. Oblique views may be needed. Seen in the 9- to 36-month age group.

Fractures of the Ankle Region (Distal Tibial Physis)

Triplane fracture of the distal tibial epiphysis: Long-term follow-up. Ertl JP, Barrack RL, Alexander AH, et al. *J Bone Joint Surg* 1988;70A:967-976.

> This article is unique in providing a relatively long-term follow-up (3 to 13 years) on an intra-articular fracture that occurs in a young person. Although symptoms were absent on early follow-up, about half of the patients were symptomatic on long-term evaluation. When the fracture extended into the weightbearing area of the ankle, residual displacement of 2 mm or more was associated with suboptimal results.

Triplane fractures of the distal tibial epiphysis. Spiegel PG, Mast JW, Cooperman DR, et al. *Clin Orthop* 1984;188:74-89.

> A follow-up on the original report of 15 cases (*J Bone Joint Surg* 1978;60A:1040-1046) of triplane fractures. This article describes in detail the pathology of the fracture fragments, diagnostic techniques, and treatment principles of this uncommon lesion. Recommends internal fixation for fracture gaps greater than 2 mm.

Distal tibial physeal fractures in children that may require open reduction. Kling TF Jr, Bright RW, Hensinger RN. *J Bone Joint Surg* 1984;66A:647-657.

> Studied fractures that most commonly lead to growth arrest. Found high incidence of growth arrest in those Salter-Harris types III and IV involving the medial malleolus (supination inversion injury) that were not anatomically reduced. For good results, recommends open reduction for most of these fracture patterns.

Pronation injuries of the ankle in children: Retrospective study of radiographical classification and treatment. Kärrholm J, Hansson LI, Laurin S. *Acta Orthop Scand* 1983;54:1-17.

> The most extensive discussion of the various types of pronation injuries in children. Describes subgroups based on the fracture pattern seen. Most common complication was periosteal interposition with a subsequent valgus deformity.

Epiphyseal fractures of the distal ends of the tibia and fibula: A retrospective study of two hundred and thirty-seven cases in children. Spiegel PG, Cooperman DR, Laros GS. *J Bone Joint Surg* 1978;60A:1046-1050.

> A report of 184 fractures reviewed for follow-up sequelae. Noted high risk for growth arrest occurred in Salter-Harris types III and IV fractures with displacement greater than 2 mm.

Physeal injuries of the ankle in children: Classification. Dias LS, Tachdjian MO. *Clin Orthop* 1978;136:230-233.
> Describes a classification modifying the Lauge-Hansen mechanism of injury principle and applies it to patients with open physes. Four major groups: supination inversion, supination plantar flexion, supination external rotation, and pronation-eversion-external rotation.

An unusual fracture of the tibial epiphysis. Marmor L. *Clin Orthop* 1970;73:132-135.
> The original description of the triplane fracture. Describes a three-part fracture pattern.

Injuries of the distal tibial epiphysis. Crenshaw AH. *Clin Orthop* 1965;41:98-107.
> One of the original fracture classifications based on the initial work of Ashurst and Bromer in 1936. Classification is by direction of deforming forces and position of the fragments after fracture.

Fracture of the lateral portion of the distal tibial epiphysis. Kleiger B, Mankin HJ. *J Bone Joint Surg* 1964;46A:25-32.
> The original description of the juvenile Tillaux fracture. Describes the early closure of the medial aspect of the physis leaving the lateral portion open in adolescence.

Varus deformity of ankle following injury to distal epiphyseal cartilage of tibia in growing children. Gill GG, Abbott LC. *Surg Gynecol Obstet* 1941;72:659-666.
> Describes the varus deformity that occurs as the result of arrest of the medial portion of the distal tibial physis with overgrowth of fibula. Details the surgical correction of this deformity.

The Foot

The blood supply of the talus. Mulfinger GL, Trueta J. *J Bone Joint Surg* 1970;52B:160-167.
> Describes the blood supply of the talus as coming from three sources. Points out the vulnerability of the neck to developing avascular necrosis in fractures.

Transchondral fractures (osteochondritis dissecans) of the talus. Berndt AL, Harty M. *J Bone Joint Surg* 1959;41A:988-1020.
> The most complete review of the types, mechanisms of injury, and treatment of this injury in the orthopaedic literature. Differentiates between medial and lateral injuries. Found that conservative management gave poor results in both children and adults. Describes four stages in these injuries.

Osteochondral lesions of the talus. Canale ST, Belding RH. *J Bone Joint Surg* 1980;62A:97-102.

> A review of 29 patients showed that lateral lesions associated with trauma were more likely to be symptomatic. Gives treatment recommendations, using Berndt and Harty classifications.

Fractures of the neck of the talus in children. Letts RM, Gibeault D. *Foot Ankle* 1980;1:74-77.

> Reports 12 cases of fractures of the talar neck in children, four of which involved children less than 3 years of age. Noted avascular necrosis in undisplaced fractures.

Calcaneal fractures in children: An evaluation of the nature of the injury in 56 children. Schmidt TL, Weiner DS. *Clin Orthop* 1982;171:150-155.

> Reviews patterns of these injuries in children. Compared with adults, children have a higher incidence of injury by lawnmower or direct blows, a higher incidence of other associated fractures, and fewer intra-articular fractures.

Tarso-metatarsal joint injuries in children. Wiley JJ. *J Pediatr Orthop* 1981;1:255-260.

> Describes three common mechanisms of injury. In the 18 cases reviewed, patterns of injury were similar in children and adults. All were treated with manipulative reduction, with or without percutaneous pin fixation. Results were uniformly good.

Bicycle spoke injuries of the foot and ankle in children: An underestimated "minor" injury. Izant RJ Jr, Rothmann BF, Frankel VH. *J Pediatr Surg* 1969;4:654-656.

> Describes the pathology of this injury and emphasizes that soft-tissue injury is the major component. The extent of the injury may not be initially apparent and there may be an associated fracture. Pathology is similar to that seen in a wringer injury in the upper extremity.

Bone and Joint Infections

Vernon Tolo, MD

Orthopaedic Infection: Diagnosis and Treatment. Gustilo RB, Gruninger RP, Tsukayama DT (eds). Philadelphia, WB Saunders, 1989.
> This up-to-date textbook deals with orthopaedic infections in both children and adults.

Bone and joint infections in children. Green NE, Edwards K. *Orthop Clin North Am* 1987;18:555-576.
> This extensive review article has 105 references and covers all areas of childhood musculoskeletal infection.

Etiology and medical management of acute suppurative bone and joint infections in pediatric patients. Jackson MA, Nelson JD. *J Pediatr Orthop* 1982;2:313-323.
> The use of oral antibiotics for septic arthritis and osteomyelitis is described in this review article, which also addresses the etiology of orthopaedic infections and special types of childhood infections of bones and joints.

Etiology

Acute hematogenous osteomyelitis: A model with trauma as an etiology. Morrissy RT, Haynes DW. *J Pediatr Orthop* 1989;9:447-456.
> Using a standardized injury model in the proximal tibial physis of rabbits, the authors demonstrated that injection of *Staphylococcus aureus* into the injured rabbits routinely resulted in osteomyelitis near the physeal-metaphyseal fracture site. Injection of similar bacteria into uninjured rabbits did not produce the same clinical or histologic picture of osteomyelitis.

Acute haematogenous osteomyelitis and septic arthritis--a single disease: An hypothesis based upon the presence of transphyseal blood vessels. Alderson M, Speers D, Emslie K, et al. *J Bone Joint Surg* 1986;68B:268-274.
> Injection of bacteria intravenously into chickens led to concurrent septic arthritis and osteomyelitis. Transphyseal blood vessels were noted histologically and implicated as the reason for these co-existent infections. Correlations with musculoskeletal infections in the human infant are suggested.

Evaluation

Technetium phosphate bone scan in the diagnosis of septic arthritis in childhood. Sundberg SB, Savage JP, Foster BK. *J Pediatr Orthop* 1989;9:579-585.
> In a series of 106 children with suspected septic arthritis, the technetium bone scan was shown to be ineffective in the accurate diagnosis of septic arthritis. Bone scans were able to detect adjacent osteomyelitis and to identify multifocal involvement, but were unable to differentiate between other causes of synovitis in the involved joint.

Nuclear imaging for musculoskeletal infections in children. Herndon WA, Alexieva BT, Schwindt ML, et al. *J Pediatr Orthop* 1985;5:343-347.
> Using technetium bone scans to assist in the diagnosis of osteomyelitis in 20 children, the authors found the scan not helpful in neonates and not as accurate in the foot as in other areas of the extremities. A careful clinical assessment and exam is more important to achieve an accurate diagnosis.

Gallium scintigraphy for diagnosis of septic arthritis and osteomyelitis in children. Borman TR, Johnson RA, Sherman FC. *J Pediatr Orthop* 1986;6:317-325.
> In 34 children with suspected musculoskeletal infection, the gallium scan was 91% accurate. Because the radiation exposure is higher with gallium than with technetium, this test should not be used routinely, but it is valuable in difficult-to-diagnose cases. "Ideal" candidates for a gallium scan are those with pelvic or spine infections or children with multifocal disease.

Miscellaneous

Primary subacute epiphyseal osteomyelitis: A report of three cases. Andrew TA, Porter K. *J Pediatr Orthop* 1985;5:155-157.
> The authors treated two of their three children with this rare form of osteomyelitis by using antibiotics and immobilization, but without surgery. Healing without apparent later sequelae was reported.

Subacute hematogenous osteomyelitis in children: A retrospective study. Roberts JM, Drummond DS, Breed AL, et al. *J Pediatr Orthop* 1982;2:249-254.
> The authors propose a radiographic classification for subacute hematogenous osteomyelitis. Of 55 consecutive children with hematogenous osteomyelitis, 33% had a subacute course with mild pain and few physical or laboratory signs of disease.

Pseudomonas infections in the foot following puncture wounds. Johanson PH. *JAMA* 1968;204;262-264.

The initial paper reporting the close association between puncture wounds of the foot and subsequent Pseudomonas infections.

Pseudomonas osteochondritis complicating puncture wounds of the foot in children: A 10-year evaluation. Jacobs RF, McCarthy RE, Elser JM. *J Infect Dis* 1989;160:657-661.
> Seventy-seven cases of proven pseudomonas osteomyelitis and/or septic arthritis following nail puncture wound were reviewed. Surgical debridement combined with antibiotic therapy for approximately seven days proved effective. Only two relapses occurred and both patients had a previously undetected septic arthritis.

Musculoskeletal infections in children: Part VII. Disk-space infection in children. Peterson HA. In Evarts CM (ed): American Academy of Orthopaedic Surgeons *Instructional Course Lectures, XXXII.* St. Louis, CV Mosby, 1983, pp 50-60.
> Thoroughly reviews the controversies surrounding the cause and treatment of diskitis and disk space infections in children.

Musculoskeletal infections in children: Part VI. Disseminated gonococcal infections and gonococcal arthritis. Green NE. In Evarts CM (ed): American Academy of Orthopaedic Surgeons *Instructional Course Lectures, XXXII.* St. Louis, CV Mosby, 1983, pp 48-50.
> Clinical features and diagnostic tests are emphasized in this review of gonococcal musculoskeletal infection, which is among the most common forms of septic arthritis seen in the teenage population.

A 10-year assessment of a controlled trial comparing debridement and anterior spinal fusion in the management of tuberculosis of the spine in patients on standard chemotherapy in Hong Kong: Eighth Report of the Medical Research Council Working Party on Tuberculosis of the Spine. *J Bone Joint Surg* 1982;64B:393-398.
> Although spinal fusion was noted earlier in the operated group, final follow-up revealed little difference between the results of these two groups of patients with tuberculosis of the spine.

Osteoarticular infections in children with sickle cell disease. Syrogiannopoulos GA, McCracken GH Jr, Nelson JD. *Pediatrics* 1986;78:1090-1096.
> Reviews the clinical presentation and treatment of 13 children with sickle cell disease and osteomyelitis or septic arthritis. Includes recommendations for management of sickle cell patients who present with fever and bone pain.

Treatment

Treatment of sequestra, pseudarthroses, and defects in the long bones of children who have chronic hematogenous osteomyelitis. Daoud A, Saighi-Bouaouina A. *J Bone Joint Surg* 1989;71A:1448-1468.

This review of 34 patients from Algeria with chronic hematogenous osteomyelitis reports the results of the authors' surgical management. The status of the periosteum of the infected bone was the most important factor in predicting the course of the disease and the most effective treatment.

Antimicrobial therapy of childhood skeletal infections. Scoles PV, Aronoff SC. *J Bone Joint Surg* 1984;66A:1487-1492.
This thorough review of the pharmacologic aspects of several types of antibiotics includes recommendations for antibiotic selection and principles of medical treatment of osteomyelitis and septic arthritis.

Acute septic arthritis in infancy and childhood. Nade S. *J Bone Joint Surg* 1983;65B:234-241.
In this review article, the author quotes the previous literature on septic arthritis and includes his own personal approach to this infection in childhood.

Outcome Studies

Long-term follow-up of infantile hip sepsis. Wopperer JM, White JJ, Gillespie R, et al. *J Pediatr Orthop* 1988;8:322-325.
Eight patients were followed for a mean of 31.5 years to assess the late results of infant hip infection. The authors suggest that the results of closed treatment were often superior to surgical reconstruction. It is recommended that high dislocations without an adequate femoral head be left untreated. Contralateral distal femoral epiphysiodesis can be performed in early adolescence to treat the leg length discrepancy.

Septic arthritis and osteomyelitis in children. Fink CW, Nelson JD. *Clin Rheum Dis* 1986;12:423-435.
Over a 25- to 30-year period, these authors have followed 591 cases of septic arthritis and 340 cases of osteomyelitis. Their experience is presented and compared with series reported in the literature.

Neuromuscular Diseases

Michael D. Sussman, MD

A Clinician's View of Neuromuscular Diseases, ed 2. Brooke MH. Baltimore, Williams & Wilkins, 1986.
> A very readable book which emphasizes pathophysiology and diagnosis of basic neuromuscular diseases as well as some of the "zebras". The comments on treatment are somewhat limited and there is no information on neuropathies. The book is exceedingly well referenced.

Muscle and Its Diseases: An Outline Primer of Basic Science and Clinical Methods. Siegel IM. Chicago, Yearbook Medical Publishers, 1986.
> This basic primer includes a section on normal muscle physiology as well as pathophysiology, diagnosis, and treatment of neuromuscular diseases. Covers neuronal diseases and neuropathies, as well as muscle diseases. A large amount of material is devoted to Duchenne muscular dystrophy.

Hereditary Sensory Motor Neuropathies (Charcot-Marie-Tooth Disease and Variants)

Diagnosis and Classification

Lower motor and primary sensory neuron diseases with peroneal muscular atrophy. I. Neurologic, genetic, and electrophysiologic findings in hereditary polyneuropathies, and II. Neurologic, genetic, and electrophysiologic findings in various neuronal degenerations. Dyck PJ, Lambert EH. *Arch Neurol* 1968;18:603-618, 619-625.
> The basic classification of neuronal diseases.

Hereditary motor and sensory neuropathies. Miller G, Vannucci RC. *Pediatr Ann* 1989;18:428-431.

Treatment

Long-term results of triple arthrodesis in Charcot-Marie-Tooth disease. Wetmore RS, Drennan JC. *J Bone Joint Surg* 1989;71A:417-422.
A long-term study of triple arthrodesis for correction of pes cavovarus in Charcot-Marie-Tooth disease. Wukich DK, Bowen JR. *J Pediatr Orthop* 1989;9:433-437.

The preceding two papers document the degenerative changes that occur in the ankle and mid foot after triple arthrodesis for foot deformity in patients with Charcot-Marie-Tooth disease. The optimal treatment of this problem still has not been defined.

Spinal Muscular Atrophy

Functional classification and orthopaedic management of spinal muscular atrophy. Evans GA, Drennan JC, Russman BS. *J Bone Joint Surg* 1981;63B:516-522.
> Fifty-four patients were reviewed for musculoskeletal problems associated with spinal muscular atrophy. Functional classification makes it possible to anticipate problems and plan treatment.

The orthopaedic aspects of spinal muscular atrophy. Schwentker EP, Gibson DA. *J Bone Joint Surg* 1976;58A:32-38.
> An excellent review of problems and management of patients with spinal muscular atrophy.

Spine fusion in patients with spinal muscular atrophy. Aprin H, Bowen JR, MacEwen GD, et al. *J Bone Joint Surg* 1982;64A:1179-1187.
Spinal deformities in patients with spinal muscle atrophy: A review of 36 patients. Riddick MF, Winter RB, Lutter LD. *Spine* 1982;7:476-483.
Spinal surgery in spinal muscular atrophy. Daher YH, Lonstein JE, Winter RB, et al. *J Pediatr Orthop* 1985;5:391-395.
> These three papers document the experience in three different centers with the surgical treatment of spinal deformity in spinal muscular atrophy. Nonambulatory patients develop severe deformities that should be treated before pulmonary function deteriorates and deformities progress to a severe magnitude. Techniques used include anterior fusion, which is not recommended because of its effects on ventilation in these patients, who are diaphragmatic breathers. Two patients in the series of Daher and associates were treated with Luque SSI--the current treatment of choice. None of the papers offers a solution for severely involved patients who develop major curvatures at a young age (4 to 6 years old). These patients are not well controlled by bracing and at that age are not good candidates for long spinal fusion.

Duchenne Muscular Dystrophy

Diagnosis, management, and orthopaedic treatment of muscular dystrophy. Siegel IM. In Murray DG (ed): American Academy of Orthopaedic Surgeons *Instructional Course Lectures, XXX*. St. Louis, CV Mosby, 1981, pp 3-35.
> This instructional course outlines the treatment used by orthopaedic pioneers to treat Duchenne Muscular Dystrophy, an approach that includes release of contractures at the hips and foot and ankle by percutaneous methods.

The orthopaedic care of children with muscular dystrophy. Green NE. In Griffin PP (ed): American Academy of Orthopaedic Surgeons *Instructional Course Lectures, XXXVI*. Park Ridge, IL, American Academy of Orthopaedic Surgeons, 1987, pp 267-274.

> Summarizes the orthopaedic management of patients with Duchenne Muscular Dystrophy.

Diagnosis and Pathophysiology

Prenatal diagnosis of Duchenne muscular dystrophy: Prospective linkage analysis and retrospective dystrophic cDNA analysis. Ward PA, Hejtmancik JF, Witkowski JA, et al. *Am J Hum Genet* 1989;44:270-281.

> Explains the use of linkage analysis to do prenatal diagnostic studies in mothers who are obligate heterozygotes.

Improved diagnosis of Becker muscular dystrophy by dystrophin testing. Hoffman EP, Kunkel LM, Angelini C, et al. *Neurology* 1989;39:1011-1017. Dystrophin abnormalities in Duchenne-Becker muscular dystrophy. Hoffman EP, Kunkel LM. *Neuron* 1989;2:1019-1029.

> These two articles describe the use of dystrophin analysis in muscle specimens in diagnosing of Duchenne and Becker Muscular Dystrophy. These techniques have also defined the basic defect in Duchenne-Becker muscular dystrophy, which is defective dystrophin synthesis in muscle of affected patients.

Delay in diagnosing Duchenne muscular dystrophy in orthopaedic clinics. Read L, Galasko CS. *J Bone Joint Surg* 1986;68B:481-482.

> Delayed diagnosis of Duchenne Muscular Dystrophy results in a delay in appropriate genetic counseling that would allow families to make informed decisions on subsequent pregnancies. In a survey of 83 families, it was found that in every case referred to an orthopaedic surgeon (37 patients), the diagnosis was missed. In general, the diagnosis was delayed by a mean of two years following initial suspicions by the family.

Nonsurgical Management

Clinical investigation of Duchenne muscular dystrophy: A methodology for therapeutic trials based on natural history controls. Mendell JR, Province MA, Moxley RT III, et al. *Arch Neurol* 1987;44:808-811.
Randomized, double-blind six-month trial of prednisone in Duchenne's muscular dystrophy. Mendell JR, Moxley RT, Griggs RC, et al. *N Engl J Med* 1989;320:1592-1597.

> The first of these two papers defines a group of clinical tests that accurately measure the loss of function with time in patients with Duchenne Muscular Dystrophy. The other paper uses these tests to demonstrate a positive effect of Prednisone in preventing the progression

of muscular weakness in patients with Duchenne Muscular Dystrophy in a six-month clinical trial.

Prevention of rapidly progressive scoliosis in Duchenne muscular dystrophy by prolongation of walking with orthoses. Rodillo EB, Fernandez-Bermejo E, Heckmatt JZ, et al. *J Child Neurol* 1988;3:269-274.
> Demonstrates a reduction in the rate of curve progression in patients who continued to ambulate in orthoses between 13 and 15 years of age, compared with a control group who ceased walking.

Ventilator management in Duchenne muscular dystrophy and postpoliomyelitis syndrome: Twelve years' experience. Curran FJ, Colbert AP. *Arch Phys Med Rehabil* 1989;70:180-185.
> Negative pressure body ventilators are recommended for partial respiratory support until the duration of respiratory support is such that a tracheostomy must be performed. The average length of survival was prolonged from 19 years and 9 months to 25 years and 9 months in patients with Duchenne Muscular Dystrophy.

Upper limb weakness in children with Duchenne muscular dystrophy: A neglected problem. James WV, Orr JF. *Prosthet Orthot* 1984;8:111-113.
> Upper limb weakness has significant impact on functional activities of patients with Duchenne muscular dystrophy. This article describes a motorized counterweight system of arm suspension that allows greater upper extremity function.

Orthopaedic Management - Extremities

Orthopaedic management of childhood neuromuscular disease: Part III. Disease of muscle. Shapiro F, Bresnan MJ. *J Bone Joint Surg* 1982;64A:1102-1107.
> A review article.

The management of equinus deformity in Duchenne muscular dystrophy. Williams EA, Read L, Ellis A, et al. *J Bone Joint Surg* 1984;66B:546-550.
> Progression of equinus deformity could not be corrected by nonsurgical means. The authors propose surgical correction for foot deformities that interfere with function.

Predicting the success of reambulation in patients with Duchenne muscular dystrophy. Vignos PJ Jr, Wagner MB, Kaplan JS, et al. *J Bone Joint Surg* 1983;65A:719-728.
> Various biochemical and clinical variables were evaluated to determine the predicted duration of continued walking following surgery and bracing in patients with Duchenne's muscular dystrophy. The most useful factors were percentage of residual muscle strength, vital capacity, creatinine coefficient, motivation of the patient, and decrease in creatinine coefficient in the two years prior to bracing.

Orthopaedic Management - Spine

Scoliosis associated with Duchenne muscular dystrophy. Cambridge W, Drennan JC. *J Pediatr Orthop* 1987;7:436-440.
> Analyzes the natural history of scoliosis, which occurred in 95% of the patient population.

Surgical stabilization of the spine in Duchenne muscular dystrophy. Weimann RL, Gibson DA, Moseley CF, et al. *Spine* 1983;8:776-780.
> The early experience with spinal stabilization using Harrington instrumentation from the upper thoracic spine to the sacrum. This technique has been superseded by Luque segmental spinal instrumentation.

Advantage of early spinal stabilization and fusion in patients with Duchenne muscular dystrophy. Sussman MD. *J Pediatr Orthop* 1984;4:532-537.
> Patients who underwent Luque instrumentation from the upper thoracic spine to L-5 had a more benign postoperative course when surgery was done in curves less than 60 degrees. Spinal bracing is ineffective in patients with Duchenne Muscular Dystrophy.

The treatment of scoliosis in Duchenne muscular dystrophy. Rideau Y, Glorion B, Delaubier A, et al. *Muscle Nerve* 1984;7:281-286.
> Prophylactic spinal fusion is recommended for all Duchenne Muscular Dystrophy patients before they experience a marked decrease in pulmonary function. To do so diminishes the risks of pulmonary complications in this group.

Arthrogryposis

The pathophysiology of arthrogryposis multiplex congenita neurologica. Brown LM, Robson MJ, Sharrard WJ. *J Bone Joint Surg* 1980;62B:291-296.
> Reviews the patterns of deformity and muscle activity in 11 patients with arthrogryposis. Based on previous studies of the spinal cord, the clinical picture was consistent with localized lesions of the anterior horn cell columns.

An approach to research on congenital contractures. Hall JG. *Birth Defects* 1984;20:8-30.
> A basic classification for arthrogryposis. Includes some information on pathophysiology and etiology based on the largest patient group in the literature.

The management of arthrogryposis. Williams P. *Orthop Clin North Am* 1978;9:67-88.
Ambulation in severe arthrogryposis. Hoffer MM, Swank S, Eastman F, et al. *J Pediatr Orthop* 1983;3:293-296.

Of 36 severely affected arthrogrypotic patients, 22 were able to achieve functional ambulation. Requirements were less than 30 degrees of hip flexion contracture, less than 20 degrees of knee flexion contracture, good hip extensor and quadriceps strength, or upper extremities strong enough to allow use of crutches. Major foot or spine deformities also diminished the likelihood of functional ambulation.

Upper Extremity

Surgical management of arthrogryposis in the upper extremity. Bennett JB, Hansen PE, Granberry WM, et al. *J Pediatr Orthop* 1985;5:281-286.
Reviews various surgical procedures used in treating arthrogryposis.

Restoration of elbow flexion in arthrogryposis multiplex congenita. Doyle JR, James PM, Larsen LJ, et al. *J Hand Surg* 1980;5:149-152.
Pectoralis major transfer for paralysis of elbow flexion in children. Atkins RM, Bell MJ, Sharrard WJ. *J Bone Joint Surg* 1985;67B:640-644.
These two papers found the pectoralis major transfer to be an effective procedure for restoration of elbow function in children with arthrogryposis.

Arthrogryposis of the hand. Yonenobu K, Tada K, Swanson AB. *J Pediatr Orthop* 1984;4:599-603.
Of 45 cases reviewed, 29 hands in 17 patients were successfully treated by surgery.

Foot and Ankle

The arthrogrypotic foot plan of management and results of treatment. Zimbler S, Craig CL. *Foot Ankle* 1983;3:211-219.
Of 51 deformed feet in this group, 40 had severe equinovarus deformity. The remainder had metatarsus adductus, vertical tali, and calcaneovalgus. Radical posteromedial release gave the best initial results. Four feet with persistent deformity were managed by talectomy.

Talectomy for arthrogryposis multiplex congenita. Green AD, Fixsen JA, Lloyd-Roberts GC. *J Bone Joint Surg* 1984;66B:697-699.
Talectomy for clubfoot in arthrogryposis. Hsu LC, Jaffray D, Leong JC. *J Bone Joint Surg* 1984;66B:694-696.
Talectomy in the treatment of resistant talipes equinovarus deformity in myelomeningocele and arthrogryposis. Dias LS, Stern LS. *J Pediatr Orthop* 1987;7:39-41.
These three papers all support talectomy as a good salvage procedure for treatment of persistent equinovarus deformity following posteromedial release in patients with arthrogryposis.

Clinical Orthopaedics and Related Research 1985; vol 194.
This volume contains 15 articles on arthrogryposis.

Spine

Scoliosis in arthrogryposis multiplex congenita. Herron LD, Westin GW, Dawson EG. *J Bone Joint Surg* 1978;60A:293-299.
Scoliosis in arthrogryposis multiplex congenita. Drummond DS, Mackenzie DA. *Spine* 1978;3:146-151.
> These two articles deal with the high incidence of scoliosis in arthrogryposis (20% to 30%). In both series the curves were long C-curves that were rigid and progressed despite bracing. Associated problems were dislocation of the hips and pelvic obliquity.

Friedreich's Ataxia

The surgical management of Friedreich's ataxia. Makin M. *J Bone Joint Surg* 1953;35A:425-436.
> A 20-year review of 45 patients with this disorder. (Some may have had forms of Charcot-Marie-Tooth disease.) Most common surgical procedure was triple arthrodesis with or without Hibbs tendon transfers. Even though the disease is progressive, surgery appeared to decrease the effects of ataxia and improve overall functional activity.

Spinal deformities in patients with Friedreich ataxia: A review of 19 patients. Daher YH, Lonstein JE, Winter RB, et al. *J Pediatr Orthop* 1985;5:553-557.
> Bracing failed to prevent curve progression in this group of 14 patients, 12 of whom came to surgery. Long paralytic "C" curve patterns were not seen, and 8 of the patients had thoracic hyperkyphosis.

Incidence, natural history, and treatment of scoliosis in Friedreich's ataxia. Cady RB, Bobechko WP. *J Pediatr Orthop* 1984;4:673-676.
> Of 32 patients who presented with complaints ultimately diagnosed as Friedrich's ataxia, 28 (88%) developed significant scoliosis. In these patients, and also in a group who presented with scoliosis, the curves tended to be progressive and unresponsive to bracing. Long-term results of surgical treatment with Harrington Rod instrumentation were good, despite one perioperative death from cardiac complication. Early spinal fusion, before the deformity becomes severe, is recommended.

Miscellaneous

Malignant hyperthermia: Current concepts. Marchildon MB. *Arch Surg* 1982;117:349-351.
> A good review of the incidence, diagnosis, theories of etiology, and treatment of anesthetic complications. Emphasizes that vigilance for this

problem needs to be especially high in patients with myopathies who are undergoing surgical procedures.

Myopathies of infancy and childhood. Miller G. *Pediatr Ann* 1989;18:439-453.

Course, prognosis and complications of childhood-onset myotonic dystrophy. O'Brien TA, Harper PS. *Dev Med Child Neurol* 1984;26:62-67.
> Neonates with myotonic dystrophy who are born of mothers with myotonic dystrophy will demonstrate severe involvement and may require early respiratory support. They do, however, have significant potential for improvement.

Thoracoscapular fusion for facioscapulohumeral dystrophy. Copeland SA, Howard RC. *J Bone Joint Surg* 1978;60B:547-551.
> Describes fusion of the scapula to the posterior ribs to prevent winging and improve upper extremity stability in patients with facioscapulohumeral dystrophy.

Cerebral Palsy

Michael D. Sussman, MD

Orthopedic Management of Cerebral Palsy. Bleck EE. Philadelphia, JB Lippincott, 1987.
> This well referenced, comprehensive text covers all aspects of cerebral palsy. It presents some of the author's biases, but most of these are well substantiated, and conflicting positions are also presented. This book should be read by all residents and practitioners who work with cerebral palsy patients.

Gait Disorders in Childhood and Adolescence. Sutherland DH. Williams & Wilkins, Baltimore, 1984.
> A basic primer on gait analysis and normal gait with a large section on gait deviations in cerebral palsy.

Antecedents of cerebral palsy: Multivariate analysis of risk. Nelson KB, Ellenberg JH. *N Engl J Med* 1986;315:81-86.
> This paper, based on a study of 54,000 pregnancies between 1959 and 1966, concludes that important predisposing factors in children born with cerebral palsy include maternal mental retardation, birth weight below 2,001 grams, fetal malformation, and breech presentation. Unexpected asphyxia in full-term infants was an unusual cause of cerebral palsy. Also see the accompanying editorial in the same issue (Birth in the origins of cerebral palsy: Paneth N, 124-126).

Locomotor prognosis in cerebral palsy. Bleck EE. *Dev Med Child Neurol* 1975;17:18-25.
> This classic paper describes a series of clinical tests that are useful predictors of long-term function. These tests also provide a basic framework for developmental assessment by the orthopaedist of children with cerebral palsy

Gait Analysis

Angle-angle diagrams in monitoring and quantification of gait patterns for children with cerebral palsy. de Bruin H, Russell DJ, Latter JE, et al. *Am J Phys Med* 1982;61:176-192.
> Offers an explanation of a data display technique.

Clinical experience of gait analysis in the management of cerebral palsy. Baumann JU. *Prosthet Orthot Int* 1984;8:29-32.

Pre- and postoperative gait analysis in patients with spastic diplegia: A preliminary report. Gage JR, Fabian D, Hicks R, et al. *J Pediatr Orthop* 1984;4:715-725.

> Explains gait analysis and shows how it is used to demonstrate changes following surgical intervention.

Energy cost index as an estimate of energy expenditure of cerebral-palsied children during assisted ambulation. Rose J, Medeiros JM, Parker R. *Dev Med Child Neurol* 1985;27:485-490.

> Heart rate is used to compare energy expenditure of children who use walkers with those using quadripod canes.

An overview of normal walking. Gage JR. In Greene WB (ed): American Academy of Orthopaedic Surgeons *Instructional Course Lectures, XXXIX*. Park Ridge, IL, American Academy of Orthopaedic Surgeons, 1990, pp 291-303.
Pathologic gait. Perry J. In Greene WB (ed): American Academy of Orthopaedic Surgeons *Instructional Course Lectures, XXXIX*. Park Ridge, IL, American Academy of Orthopaedic Surgeons, 1990, pp 325-331.
Gait analysis in neuromuscular diseases. Sutherland DH. In Greene WB (ed): American Academy of Orthopaedic Surgeons *Instructional Course Lectures, XXXIX*. Park Ridge, IL, American Academy of Orthopaedic Surgeons, 1990, pp 333-341.

> These three articles, which describe in significant detail the kinematics of normal walking, pathologic gait, and gait analysis in cerebral palsy, are basic reading for orthopaedic surgery residents and for any orthopaedic surgeon taking care of children with cerebral palsy.

Nonsurgical Treatment

Accepted and controversial neuromotor therapies for infants at high risk for cerebral palsy. Harris SR, Atwater SW, Crowe TK. *J Perinatol* 1988;8:3-13.

> Assesses therapies for high-risk patients.

The effects of physical therapy on cerebral palsy: A controlled trial in infants with spastic diplegia. Palmer FB, Shapiro BK, Wachtel RC, et al. *N Engl J Med* 1988;318:803-808.

> This well designed study compared six months of neurodevelopmental therapy with a cognitively based stimulation program. The infants in the neurodevelopment treatment therapy program did not perform as well as those in the infant stimulation program. This is one of the best studies on the efficacy of physical therapy.

A review of therapeutic intervention research on gross and fine motor progress in young children with cerebral palsy. Parette HP Jr, Hourcade JJ. *Am J Occup Ther* 1984;38:462-468.
Foot reflexes and the use of the "inhibitive cast". Duncan WR, Mott DH. *Foot Ankle* 1983;4:145-148.

Effect of short leg casting on ambulation in children with cerebral palsy. Bertoti DB. *Phys Ther* 1986;66:1522-1529.

A prospective study of inhibitive casting as an adjunct to physiotherapy for cerebral-palsied children. Watt J, Sims D, Harckham F, et al. *Dev Med Child Neurol* 1986;28:480-488.

> These four studies explain the theory and attempt to demonstrate the efficacy of "inhibitive casting" for children with cerebral palsy. Arguments for this approach, however, remain unconvincing.

The use of orthotics in foot and ankle problems in cerebral palsy. Rosenthal RK. *Foot Ankle* 1984;4:195-200.

> Appropriate molding can correct balance, stance phase, and swing-phase difficulties, and can also be used to control dynamic muscle imbalances.

The Doman-Delacato treatment of neurologically handicapped children: Policy statement. American Academy of Pediatrics. *Pediatrics* 1982;70:810-812.

> This policy statement concludes that there is no strong evidence for the efficacy of the Doman-Delacato method for treating cerebral palsy.

Sitting problems of children with cerebral palsy. Fulford GE, Cairns TP, Sloan Y. *Dev Med Child Neurol* 1982;24:48-53.

Seating for children with cerebral palsy. Rang M, Douglas G, Bennet GC, et al. *J Pediatr Orthop* 1981;1:279-287.

Early physiotherapy in the treatment of spastic diplegia. Kanda T, Yuge M, Yamori Y, et al. *Dev Med Child Neurol* 1984;26:438-444.

Electromyographic investigation of extensor activity in cerebral-palsied children in different seating positions. Nwaobi OM, Brubaker CE, Cusick B, et al. *Dev Med Child Neurol* 1983;25:175-183.

> The preceding 4 papers address the important subject of seating for patients with cerebral palsy. The paper by Nwaobi uses quantitative electromyelography to compare different seating positions.

Muscle growth in normal and spastic mice. Ziv I, Blackburn N, Rang M, et al. *Dev Med Child Neurol* 1984;26:94-99.

> Demonstrates that muscle growth, which occurs at the musculotendinous junction, is impaired in spastic mice, resulting in contracture.

Surgery - Reviews and Principles

Static and dynamic problems in spastic cerebral palsy. Reimers J. *J Bone Joint Surg* 1973;55B:822-827.

> This classic paper, which outlines principles of surgical treatment for patients with cerebral palsy, is still relevant.

Cerebral palsy: The first three years. Hoffer MM, Koffman M. *Clin Orthop* 1980;151:222-227.

> During the first three years of life, surgical treatment for cerebral palsy is usually limited to adductor releases about the hip. Stretching, plaster

splints about the knee and ankle, and ankle-foot orthoses can help correct deformity.

Current concepts of surgical management of deformities of the lower extremities in cerebral palsy. Samilson RL. *Clin Orthop* 1981;158:99-107.
One-session surgery for correction of lower extremity deformities in children with cerebral palsy. Norlin R, Tkaczuk H. *J Pediatr Orthop* 1985;5:208-211.
One-session surgery for bilateral correction of lower limb deformities in spastic diplegia. Browne AO, McManus F. *J Pediatr Orthop* 1987;7:259-261.
> The preceding papers reflect the current consensus regarding surgery-- that deformities in the lower extremities are linked and should be corrected simultaneously to allow more effective rehabilitation.

Assessment and management of the lower extremity in cerebral palsy. Jones ET, Knapp DR. *Orthop Clin North Am* 1987;18:725-738.
> Early aggressive treatment to achieve muscle balancing will facilitate function and reduce the risk of bone deformity.

The orthopaedic management of the ankle, foot, and knee in patients with cerebral palsy. Green NE. In Griffin PP (ed): American Academy of Orthopaedic Surgeons *Instructional Course Lectures, XXXVI*. Park Ridge, IL, American Academy of Orthopaedic Surgeons, 1987, pp 253-265.
> Stresses importance of evaluating all problems in children with cerebral palsy before undertaking surgical treatment.

Hip - General

Treatment of hip problems in cerebral palsy. Root L. In Griffin PP (ed): American Academy of Orthopaedic Surgeons *Instructional Course Lectures, XXXVI*. Park Ridge, IL, American Academy of Orthopaedic Surgeons, 1987, pp 237-252.
> Treatment options for the spastic dysplastic hip include total hip replacement and fusion.

Natural history of the dislocated hip in spastic cerebral palsy. Moreau M, Drummond DS, Rogala E, et al. *Dev Med Child Neurol* 1979;21:749-753.
> Reviews 88 adult, institutionalized cerebral palsy patients.

The untreated unstable hip in severe cerebral palsy. Pritchett JW. *Clin Orthop* 1983;173:169-172.
> Reviews 80 institutionalized patients, both adults and children, with subluxed or dislocated hips. Direction of scoliosis, pelvic obliquity, and side of hip dislocation correlated in most patients.

Management of the hip in cerebral palsy. Hoffer MM. *J Bone Joint Surg* 1986;68A:629-631.
> Reviews current concepts. Well referenced.

Hip dislocation in spastic cerebral palsy: Long-term consequences. Cooperman DR, Bartucci E, Dietrick E, et al. *J Pediatr Orthop* 1987;7:268-276.

> Reviews 38 non-institutionalized spastic quadriplegic patients with 51 dislocated hips, 9 of which had been reduced. Authors recommend reduction of all uni- and bilateral dislocations if femoral head deformity is not present.

Hip - Adductor Surgery

Dislocation of the hip in cerebral palsy: Natural history and predictability. Cooke PH, Cole WG, Carey RPL. *J Bone Joint Surg* 1989;71B:441-446.

> The authors determined that acetabular index, when corrected for pelvic rotation, was one of the most powerful predictors of ultimate hip dislocation.

The stability of the hip in children: A radiological study of the results of muscle surgery in cerebral palsy. Reimers J. *Acta Orthop Scand* 1980;184(suppl):1-100.

> In this large study, the author concludes that the migration percentage is the most effective technique for measuring hip dysplasia. Demonstrates the efficacy of adductor muscle surgery and notes factors that can influence the ultimate result.

Adductor tenotomy-obturator neurectomy. Wheeler ME, Weinstein SL. *J Pediatr Orthop* 1984;4:48-51.

> Demonstrates effectiveness of this procedure through a 3.7-year follow-up of 25 cerebral palsy patients.

Adductor release in nonambulant children with cerebral palsy. Silver RL, Rang M, Chan J, et al. *J Pediatr Orthop* 1985;5:672-677.

> Adductor release prevented hip dislocation in 80% of 50 non-ambulatory patients. Failure rate was highest when uncoverage exceeded 50%.

Prevention of spastic paralytic dislocation of the hip. Kalen V, Bleck EE. *Dev Med Child Neurol* 1985;27:17-24.

> Notes the positive effects of recessing the iliopsoas at the time of adductor releases.

Treatment of acquired hip subluxation in cerebral palsy. Houkom JA, Roach JW, Wenger DR, et al. *J Pediatr Orthop* 1986;6:285-290.

> The results following adductor release surgery can be improved by long-term use of sleeping orthoses.

Hip - Bony Surgery

Hip adductor transfer compared with adductor tenotomy in cerebral palsy. Root L, Spero CR. *J Bone Joint Surg* 1981;63A:767-772.
Adductor transfer versus tenotomy for stability of the hip in spastic cerebral palsy. Reimers J, Poulsen S. *J Pediatr Orthop* 1984;4:52-54.
> The preceding two papers discuss adductor transfer as an alternative to adductor tenotomy. The paper by Root and associates demonstrates that adductor transfer is more effective than adductor tenotomy; the other study found no significant difference.

Proximal femoral osteotomy in cerebral palsy. Tylkowski CM, Rosenthal RK, Simon SR. *Clin Orthop* 1980;151:183-192.
Femoral varus-derotation osteotomy in spastic cerebral palsy. Hoffer MM, Stein GA, Koffman M, et al. *J Bone Joint Surg* 1985;67A:1229-1235.
> These two papers demonstrate the efficacy of proximal femoral osteotomy for treatment of hip dysplasia that did not respond to adductor muscle release.

Slotted acetabular augmentation. Staheli LT. *J Pediatr Orthop* 1981;1:321-327.
> Technique of performing acetabular shelf.

Proximal femoral resection-interposition arthroplasty. Castle ME, Schneider C. *J Bone Joint Surg* 1978;60A:1051-1054.
> Subsequent studies have confirmed that Castle's procedure is effective in achieving mobility and diminishing pain in patients with established painful dislocation of the hip in cerebral palsy.

Total hip replacement in young people with neurological disease. Root L. *Dev Med Child Neurol* 1982;24:186-188.
> Presents another approach for the salvage of the painful total hip dislocation in the spastic patient. Indications are limited.

Supracondylar derotational osteotomy of the femur for internal rotation of the thigh in the cerebral palsied child. Hoffer MM, Prietto C, Koffman M. *J Bone Joint Surg* 1981;63A:389-393.
> Presents a technique for femoral derotation osteotomy that will allow early ambulation.

The Windblown Hip

The windblown hip syndrome in total body cerebral palsy. Letts M, Shapiro L, Mulder K, et al. *J Pediatr Orthop* 1984;4:55-62.
> Demonstrates that hip adduction and dysplasia precede pelvic obliquity and scoliosis in cases where these entities co-exist.

Hip dislocation and subluxation in cerebral palsy. Lonstein JE, Beck K. *J Pediatr Orthop* 1986;6:521-526.

These authors were unable to demonstrate a relationship between hip subluxation, pelvic obliquity, and scoliosis.

Knee

Distal hamstring lengthening in cerebral palsy: An evaluation by gait analysis. Baumann JU, Ruetsch H, Schurmann K. *Int Orthop* 1980;3:305-309.
> Results of long-term follow-up of 34 patients.

A long-term retrospective study of proximal hamstring release for hamstring contracture in cerebral palsy. Sharps CH, Clancy M, Steel HH. *J Pediatr Orthop* 1984;4:443-447.
> Of 78 patients, 32 were assessed at a mean of nine years and five months after surgery. Of 64 knees, only 4 were in mild recurvatum. Lumbar lordosis rate was 55%.

The effect on gait of lengthening of the medial hamstrings in cerebral palsy. Thometz J, Simon S, Rosenthal R. *J Bone Joint Surg* 1989;71A:345-353.
> Although stance-phase knee extension improved, swing-phase knee flexion diminished following hamstring-lengthening surgery.

Rectus femoris transfer to improve knee function of children with cerebral palsy. Gage JR, Perry J, Hicks RR, et al. *Dev Med Child Neurol* 1987;29:159-166.
> In cerebral patients with hamstring spasticity, the rectus femoris often has dysphasic terminal stance and swing activity while it is silent in stance phase. In these patients, when the rectus femoris was transferred to the distal stump of the hamstrings at the time of hamstring lengthening, patients demonstrated improved stance-phase knee extension along with improved swing-phase knee flexion.

Recurvatum

A fixed-ankle, below-the-knee orthosis for the management of genu recurvatum in spastic cerebral palsy. Rosenthal RK, Deutsch SD, Miller W, et al. *J Bone Joint Surg* 1975;57A:545-547.
> Describes a floor reaction ankle-foot orthosis for treatment of mild recurvatum in patients with cerebral palsy. This molded plastic orthosis is fabricated with the foot in 5 to 10 degrees of dorsiflexion. The floor reaction force restrains the knee from progressing into recurvatum.

Genu recurvatum in spastic cerebral palsy: Report on findings by gait analysis. Simon SR, Deutsch SD, Nuzzo RM, et al. *J Bone Joint Surg* 1978;60A:882-894.
> Limitation of mid-stance dorsiflexion appears to be the major determinant of genu recurvatum during walking.

Foot and Ankle Equinus

Equinus and cerebral palsy--its management. Banks HH. *Foot Ankle* 1983;4:149-159.

Calcaneus deformity in cerebral palsy. Dillin W, Samilson RL. *Foot Ankle* 1983;4:167-170.

Calcaneal gait in spastic diplegia after heel cord lengthening: A study with gait analysis. Segal LS, Sienko Thomas SE, Mazur JM, et al. *J Pediatr Orthop* 1989;9:697-701.
> Calcaneus deformity following Achilles tendon lengthening may be more frequent than previously recognized.

A systematic approach to the amount of Achilles tendon lengthening in cerebral palsy. Gaines RW, Ford TB. *J Pediatr Orthop* 1984;4:448-451.
> Outlines a technique for determining the amount of lengthening to be performed.

Achilles tendon lengthening in cerebral palsy: Comparison of inpatient versus ambulatory surgery. Greene WB. *J Pediatr Orthop* 1987;7:256-258.
> Describes outpatient heelcord lengthening surgery. In matched groups, outpatient heelcord lengthening was preferred because it facilitated postoperative management.

Heelcord advancement for treatment of equinus deformity in cerebral palsy. Strecker WB, Via MW, Oliver SK, et al. *J Pediatr Orthop* 1990;10:105-108.
> The technique of heelcord advancement for Achilles contracture and/or overactivity reduces the risk of overlengthening and subsequent calcaneus deformity.

Foot and Ankle - Varus/Valgus

A comparison of foot-switch and EMG analysis of varus deformities of the feet of children with cerebral palsy. Wills CA, Hoffer MM, Perry J. *Dev Med Child Neurol* 1988;30:227-231.
> Foot-switch analysis, a relatively simple technique, cannot discriminate between tibialis posterior and tibialis anterior dysfunction as the primary cause of varus deformity. Electromyographic analysis discriminates seven patterns of abnormal anterior tibialis and/or posterior tibialis activity producing varus deformity during walking. The authors do not believe that clinical examination of this problem can be done with precision.

Ten-year follow-up of split anterior tibial tendon transfer in cerebral palsied patients with spastic equinovarus deformity. Hoffer MM, Barakat G, Koffman M. *J Pediatr Orthop* 1985;5:432-434.

The split anterior tibial tendon transfer has withstood the test of time as an effective operation for treatment of the spastic varus foot, particularly when dysplastic tibialis anterior activity can be documented before surgery by electromyography.

Split posterior tibial-tendon transfer in spastic cerebral palsy. Green NE, Griffin PP, Shiavi R. *J Bone Joint Surg* 1983;65A:748-754.
   The split posterior tibial-tendon transfer has proven quite effective in the treatment of varus foot. This procedure has been used by the authors and by others without preliminary gait analysis.

Posterior tibial-tendon transfer in patients with cerebral palsy. Root L, Miller SR, Kirz P. *J Bone Joint Surg* 1987;69A:1133-1139.
   Fifty-seven posterior tibial transfers to the dorsum of the foot through the interosseous membrane into the lateral cuneiform were done in 51 patients and followed for a mean of 9.3 years. A good or excellent result was achieved in 27 of 30 feet in hemiplegic patients, 12 of 16 feet in diplegic patients, and 2 of 11 feet in spastic quadriplegic patients.

Foot and Ankle - Miscellaneous

Forefoot problems in cerebral palsy: Diagnosis and management. Bleck EE. *Foot Ankle* 1984:4:188-194.
   Forefoot problems include cavus, metatarsus adductus, hallux valgus, and bunion, dorsal bunion, and toe flexion contractures. Both prevention and correction of these deformities are surgical. Some are prevented and corrected by surgical tenotomy of the spastic muscle that causes the dynamic deformity and will eventually cause a bony abnormality. Fixed skeletal deformities need osteotomies and arthrodesis of the bones in addition to removal of the force of the deforming muscle.

Triple arthrodesis by inlay grafting: A method suitable for the undeformed or valgus foot. Williams PF, Menelaus MB. *J Bone Joint Surg* 1977;59B:333-336.
   Presents a new technique to achieve triple arthrodesis and concludes that this was an excellent procedure in a 4.5-year follow-up of 25 feet in 20 patients. Of 18 patients who were ambulatory preoperatively, three became non-ambulatory and three became brace independent.

Triple arthrodesis for children with spastic cerebral palsy. Ireland ML, Hoffer M. *Dev Med Child Neurol* 1985;27:623-627.

Spinal Deformity - Incidence and Natural History

Scoliosis in the institutionalized cerebral palsy population. Madigan RR, Wallace SL. *Spine* 1981;6:583-590.

Of 272 institutionalized patients, 64% had spinal curves greater than 10 degrees.

Progression of scoliosis after skeletal maturity in institutionalized adults who have cerebral palsy. Thometz JG, Simon SR. *J Bone Joint Surg* 1988;70A:1290-1296.
> This study documents that institutionalized cerebral palsy patients with curves that exceed 40 degrees have a high risk of progression to severe deformity.

Cervical radiculopathy or myelopathy secondary to athetoid cerebral palsy. Fuji T, Yonenobu K, Fujiwara K, et al. *J Bone Joint Surg* 1987;69A:815-821.
> Ten adult patients with athetoid cerebral palsy required surgical treatment consisting of discectomy, osteophytic removal and anterior fusion for cervical radicalopathy and/or myelopathy.

Spinal Deformity - Treatment

Interspinous process segmental spinal instrumentation for scoliosis in cerebral palsy. Sponseller PD, Whiffen JR, Drummond DS. *J Pediatr Orthop* 1986;6:559-563.
> The interspinous segmental spinal instrumentation system combined with a Harrington rod was effective in obtaining and maintaining correction of spinal deformity in patients with cerebral palsy.

L-rod instrumentation for scoliosis in cerebral palsy. Allen BL Jr, Ferguson RL. *J Pediatr Orthop* 1982;2:87-96.
Operative treatment of spinal deformities in patients with cerebral palsy or mental retardation: An analysis of one hundred and seven cases. Lonstein JE, Akbarnia A. *J Bone Joint Surg* 1983;65A:43-55.
Considerations in the treatment of cerebral palsy patients with spinal deformities. Ferguson RL, Allen BL Jr. *Orthop Clin North Am* 1988;19:419-425.
The treatment of scoliosis in cerebral palsy by posterior spinal fusion with Luque-rod segmental instrumentation. Gersoff WK, Renshaw TS. *J Bone Joint Surg* 1988;70A:41-44.
> The preceding papers all demonstrate the efficacy of the Luque technique for surgical correction and stabilization of spinal deformities in cerebral palsy. The paper by Gersoff and Renshaw includes a significant portion of patients who were fused to L-5 at the lowest level without inclusion of the sacrum.

Management of neuromuscular spinal deformities with Luque segmental instrumentation. Boachie-Adjei O, Lonstein JE, Winter RB, et al. *J Bone Joint Surg* 1989;71A:548-562.
> Reviews experience with 24 patients with cerebral palsy and 24 with other neuromuscular diseases.

Upper Extremity

Surgery of the spastic hand in cerebral palsy: Report of the Committee on Spastic Hand Evaluation (International Federation of Societies for Surgery of the Hand). Zancolli EA, Goldner LJ, Swanson AB. *J Hand Surg* 1983;8:766-772.
Management of the upper extremity in cerebral palsy. Skoff H, Woodbury DF. *J Bone Joint Surg* 1985;67A:500-503.
Surgery of the hand in cerebral palsy and muscle origin release procedures. Swanson AB. *Surg Clin North Am* 1968;48:1129-1138.
Operative treatment of cerebral palsy. Szabo RM, Gelberman RH. *Hand Clin* 1985;1:525-543.
> In these four papers, decision making is the most important factor leading to success in these procedures.

Thumb-in-Palm Deformity

Surgical treatment of spastic "thumb-in-palm" deformity. Matev I. *J Bone Joint Surg* 1963;45B:703-708.
> This progressive approach to the spastic thumb-in-palm uses an adductor origin release.

Adduction contracture of the thumb in cerebral palsy: A preoperative electromyographic study. Hoffer MM, Perry J, Garcia M, et al. *J Bone Joint Surg* 1983;65A:755-759.
> Gives treatment and results in a 23-patient study.

A dynamic approach to the thumb-in-palm deformity in cerebral palsy. House JH, Gwathmey FW, Fidler MO. *J Bone Joint Surg* 1981;63A:216-225.
> The authors report on 56 patients with cerebral palsy who underwent surgical procedures to correct thumb-in-palm deformities. Discusses indications for upper extremity surgery in cerebral palsy. Includes a classification system for thumb-in-palm deformity.

The brachioradialis for restoration of abduction and extension of spastic thumb in children. Lee BS, Horstmann H. *Orthopedics* 1984;7:1445-1558.
> Demonstrates improvement in abduction and extension of the thumb following transfer of the brachioradialis along with appropriate releases.

Wrist Flexion/Ulnar Deviation Deformity

Flexor carpi ulnaris transplant and its use in cerebral palsy. Green WT, Banks HH. *J Bone Joint Surg* 1962;44A:1343-1352.
> Describes the Green transfer of the flexor carpal ulnaris to the extensor carpi radialis brevis.

Long-term follow-up on tendon transfers to the extensors of the wrist and fingers in patients with cerebral palsy. Hoffer MM, Lehman M, Mitani M. *J Hand Surg* 1986;11A:836-840.

> Of 38 patients undergoing tendon transfers to improve wrist extension, 10 who had the worst preoperative function failed to improve while the other 28 improved. In 5 of 12 patients undergoing transfers to the wrist extensors, a wrist extension contracture developed. All of the 17 patients who had transfers to the finger extensors had improved release and no loss of grasp.

Upper extremity tendon transfers in cerebral palsy: Electromyographic and functional analysis. Mowery CA, Gelberman RH, Rhoades CE. *J Pediatr Orthop* 1985;5:69-72.

> Four of 16 transferred muscles changed phase post transfer, although all patients were clinically improved.

Treatment of pronation contractures of the forearm in cerebral palsy by changing the insertion of the pronator radii teres. Sakellarides HT, Mital MA, Lenzi WD. *J Bone Joint Surg* 1981;63A:645-652.

> Technique involves transfer of the pronator teres tendon insertion to the opposite side of the radius to act as supinator. Indications include satisfactory sensation and stereognosis, intelligence (IQ 70 or greater), and proper home environment. Forty-five degrees of passive supination is desirable, but not necessary. Postoperative average gain in supination was 46 degrees, producing a good-to-excellent result in 82%. There was no loss of supination or any function present prior to surgery. The only complications, two fractured radii, caused the technique to be changed so that the tendon was drawn through only one cortex.

Transfer of the flexor carpi ulnaris to the radial wrist extensors in cerebral palsy. Wenner SM, Johnson KA. *J Hand Surg* 1988;13A:231-233.

> Follow-up of patients undergoing the Green transfer showed improved function in most patients.

Rhizotomy

Posterior rhizotomies for spasticity in children affected by cerebral palsy. Benedetti A, Colombo F, Alexandre A, et al. *J Neurosurg Sci* 1982;26:179-184.

> An early paper on selective dorsal rhizotomy for cerebral palsy. The series includes three spastic quadriparaplegic patients who underwent upper cervical rhizotomies.

Cerebral palsy spasticity: Selective posterior rhizotomy. Peacock WJ, Arens LJ, Berman B. *Pediatr Neurosci* 1987;13:61-66.
Selective posterior rhizotomy: A long-term follow-up study. Arens LJ, Peacock WJ, Peter J. *Childs Nerv Syst* 1989;5:148-152.

The preceding two papers present the rationale, technique, and results of selective dorsal rhizotomy for the treatment of patients with cerebral palsy. Since its introduction by Peacock, whose original series was performed in South Africa, this procedure has come into relatively widespread use in this country.

Myelomeningocele

Walter B. Greene, MD

Results of treatment of myelomeningocele: An analysis of 524 unselected cases, with special reference to possible selection for treatment. Lorber J. *Dev Med Child Neurol* 1971;13:279-303.
> This article, probably one of the most controversial and oft-quoted on the subject, gives the author's perceptions on the results of 524 cases. He concludes that early selection for treatment is more humanitarian and lists criteria for selection.

Life with spina bifida. Zachary RB. *Br Med J* 1977;2:1460-1462.
> A discussion of Lorber's approach by his former neurosurgical colleagues.

Management of the newborn with myelomeningocele: Time for a decision-making process. Charney EB, Weller SC, Sutton LN, et al. *Pediatrics* 1985;75:58-64.
> Early versus delayed versus late closure of myelomeningocele defects were compared in 110 newborns. Early surgery was within the first 48 hours, delayed occurred at 3 to 7 days of age, and late closure was done 1 week to 10 months of age. Survival rates were similar in all three groups. No significant association between time of surgery and development of ventriculitis, developmental delay, or worsening of paralysis.

Influence of prognosis on decisions regarding the care of newborns with myelodysplasia. McLaughlin JF, Shurtleff DB, Lamers JY, et al. *New Engl J Med* 1985;312:1589-1594.
> Two hundred twelve newborns with myelomeningocele demonstrated improved survival with early closure whether they were classified as having a good or poor prognosis.

Impact of an intermittent catheterization program on children with myelomeningocele. Uehling DT, Smith J, Meyer J, et al. *Pediatrics* 1985;76:892-895.
> In 53 children on intermittent catheterization program for five years or more, 81% were dry, and 15% were incontinent at night only. Frequency of urinary tract infection was decreased and renal status was improved.

Myelomeningocele: Part I. General concepts. Bunch WH, pp 61-65; Part II. Management of neonatal myelomeningocele, Drennan JC, pp 65-70; Part III.

Development of the infant with myelomeningocele, Hostler SL, pp 70-75; Part IV. Treatment of the lower extremity in children paralyzed by myelomeningocele (birth to 18 months), Lindseth RE, pp 76-82; Part V. Management of myelomeningocele foot deformities in infancy and early childhood, Drennan JC, pp 82-90; Part VI. The adolescent with myelomeningocele, Hostler SL, pp 90-93; and Part VII. Treatment of the myelomeningocele spine, Bunch WH, pp 93-95. In American Academy of Orthopaedic Surgeons *Instructional Course Lectures XXV*. St. Louis, CV Mosby, 1976, pp 61-95.

> A seven-part chapter contributed by recognized experts on myelomeningocele. Some concepts are now outdated, but this review article remains a valuable reference.

The orthopaedic surgery of spina bifida. Sharrard WJW. *Clin Orthop* 1973;92:195-213.

> This pioneer in the development of orthopaedic treatment for myelomeningocele outlines his treatment program on an anatomic basis. All orthopaedic surgeons should be very knowledgeable concerning Figure 1 in this article.

Growth of trunk and legs of children with myelomeningocele. Duval-Beaupère G, Kaci M, Lougovoy J, et al. *Dev Med Child Neurol* 1987;29:225-231.

> Altered growth, as measured by an increased upper segment/lower segment ratio, was found in 78 children with myelomeningocele. The higher the level of the meningocele, the greater the effect on growth. It was concluded that neurological loss was mainly responsible for the defective growth.

The significance of spasticity in the upper and lower limbs in myelomeningocele. Mazur JM, Stillwell A, Menelaus M. *J Bone Joint Surg* 1986;68B:213-217.

> In 109 children, 54% had the expected flaccid paralysis in the lower limbs with normal upper extremities, 24% were spastic in the lower extremities but had normal upper extremities, 9% had flaccid lower limbs but spastic upper extremities, and 13% were spastic in both upper and lower extremities. Spasticity affected treatment and functional prognosis.

Hand function in patients with spina bifida cystica. Mazur JM, Menelaus MB, Hudson I, et al. *J Pediatr Orthop* 1986;6:442-447.

> One hundred forty-three patients with myelomeningocele demonstrated impaired hand function on the Jebsen-Taylor test. Thoracic and high lumbar level patients exhibited poorer hand function than low lumbar and sacral level patients. Recognition of such defects enables orthopaedic surgeons, therapists, parents, and educators to establish realistic goals for these children.

Hand function in children with myelomeningocele. Turner A. *J Bone Joint Surg* 1985;67B:268-272.

In 33 patients with myelomeningocele, the average score for hand function was 59% of normal, and only 2 children had clinically normal upper limbs. The authors did not find hand function to be better in those with lower lesions.

Magnetic resonance imaging of postrepair-myelomeningocele: Findings in 31 children and adolescents. Just M, Ermert J, Higer HP, et al. *Neurosurg Rev* 1987;10:47-52.

In 31 children who had undergone early closure of myelomeningocele, 89% had radiologic evidence of a tethered spinal cord. Progressive neurological symptoms, however, were rarely observed.

Magnetic resonance evaluation of pediatric spinal dysraphism. Kharik MA, Edwards MK, Grossman CB. *Pediatr Neurosci* 1985-86;12:213-2186.

Magnetic resonance scans of the cervicothoracic spine in 12 cases revealed 10 Chiari II malformations, 1 Chiari III malformation, and 4 syringohydromyelias. Twelve magnetic resonance imaging scans of the lumbosacral region demonstrated 11 tethered cords, 4 lypomyeloschises, 2 diastematomyelias, 2 syringohydromyelias, and 2 dermal sinus tracts.

Intraspinal rhizotomy and distal cordectomy in patients with myelomeningocele. McLaughlin TP, Banta JV, Gahm NH, et al. *J Bone Joint Surg* 1986;68A:88-94.

Intraspinal rhizotomy alone or in combination with distal cordectomy was helpful in 13 myelomeningocele patients in whom reflex spasticity caused recurrent deformity of the lower extremities. The procedure did not improve the status of the urinary tract.

Fractures

Fractures in patients who have myelomeningocele. Lock TR, Aronson DD. *J Bone Joint Surg* 1989;71A:1153-1157.

Fractures are common in children with myelomeningocele, and the incidence is related to the level of neurologic involvement. Of 76 fractures, 58 were judged to be secondary to cast immobilization. Metaphyseal and diaphyseal fractures healed satisfactorily, but the physeal plate fractures were often complicated by delayed union or premature growth arrest.

Physeal widening in children with myelomeningocele. Roberts JA, Bennet GC, MacKenzie JR. *J Bone Joint Surg* 1989;71B:30-32.

Five cases of physeal widening in children with myelomeningocele demonstrated rapid clinical resolution with minor limitation of activity. The authors suggest that recognition of the pathologic process before fracture had occurred explained the rapid return to normal.

Lower extremity fractures simulating infection in myelomeningocele. Townsend PF, Cowell HR, Steg NL. *Clin Orthop* 1979;144:255-259.

Fourteen of 33 fractures in children with myelomeningocele were accompanied by increased local heat, swelling, redness, and a systemic response including an elevated temperature and leukocyte count. Stress films may be necessary to demonstrate a suspected fracture in these patients. With proper immobilization the leukocyte count and temperature quickly return to normal.

Fractures of the lower extremities in paraplegic children. Drennan JC, Freehafer AA. *Clin Orthop* 1971;77:211-217.

Twenty-five of 84 myelomeningocele patients sustained at least one fracture of the lower extremity. The authors document the level of fracture and typical presentation for these injuries. They advocate short periods of cast immobilization and early return to braces for standing and walking activities.

Ambulation

Functional ambulation in patients with myelomeningocele. Hoffer MM, Feiwell E, Perry R, et al. *J Bone Joint Surg* 1973;55A:137-148.

Fifty-six patients were analyzed for walking status. The most important factors were level of paraplegia, central nervous system or renal anomalies, intelligence and home environment. A functional classification of ambulation (community, household, non-functional or therapy, and non-ambulators), first described in this report has been frequently used in other studies.

Factors affecting the ambulatory status of patients with spina bifida cystica. Asher M, Olson J. *J Bone Joint Surg* 1983;65A:350-356.

In a detailed assessment 16 different factors were analyzed to determine their effect on the ambulatory status of 98 myelomeningocele patients. Level of neurologic involvement was the single most significant factor. Age, obesity, and some musculoskeletal deformities were other significant variables. Different musculoskeletal deformities were important at different neurologic levels.

Walking ability in mature patients with spina bifida. Stillwell A, Menelaus MB. *J Pediatr Orthop* 1983;3:184-190.

Thirty-six of 50 adult myelomeningocele patients were able to walk. The percent walking in each group were: thoracic, 33%; high lumbar, 30%; low lumbar, 95%; and sacral, 100%. This is the only study to date which reports ambulation success in adult thoracic level patients. Negative factors for walking were severe hip flexion deformity, pelvic obliquity, and scoliosis--either alone or in combination.

Ambulation in the adolescent with myelomeningocele: I. Early childhood predictors. Findley TW, Agre JC, Habeck RV, et al. *Arch Phys Med Rehabil* 1987;68:518-522.

Seventy-seven adolescent myelomeningocele children (age 10 to 15) were assessed for ambulation ability. The ability to walk outdoors independently by age 7 was the strongest predictor of ambulation skills as an adolescent. In those who showed decreased walking during the teenage years, the beginning of the decline was associated with a period of immobilization.

Ambulation in the adolescent with spina bifida: II. Oxygen cost of mobility. Findley TW, Agre JC. *Arch Phys Med Rehabil* 1988;69:855-861.

Energy cost (measured as oxygen use) of walking and wheelchair propulsion was analyzed in adolescent children with myelomeningocele. Energy consumption for walking was linearly related to speed, slope of incline, heart rate, and body weight. For wheelchair propulsion, energy consumption was a linear function of speed, slope of incline, and body weight. Simple clinical measurements of maximum ambulatory velocity and heart rate allowed accurate prediction of energy consumption, regardless of neurologic and functional level.

Energy cost of paraplegic locomotion. Waters RL, Lunsford BR. *J Bone Joint Surg* 1985;67A:1245-1250.

One hundred fifty-one individuals with paraplegia from spinal cord injury were evaluated to determine energy expenditure during locomotion. Patients using bilateral long leg braces had an average rate of oxygen consumption that was 38% greater than that required for normal walking, and 43% greater than that of wheelchair locomotion. Patients who walked with short leg braces and crutch assistance had oxygen consumption that was 15% greater than that required for normal walking. The authors recommend that physicians emphasize to patients that reliance on a wheelchair does not constitute failure.

Energy cost of walking and of wheelchair propulsion by children with myelodysplasia: Comparison with normal children. Williams LO, Anderson AD, Campbell J, et al. *Dev Med Child Neurol* 1983;25:617-624.

Oxygen consumption during walking and propelling a wheelchair were measured in 15 myelomeningocele children. A swing-through gait pattern was 33% more energy efficient than a 4-point gait pattern. Wheelchair produced velocities and energy efficiency similar to walking by normal children.

Ambulation in patients with myelomeningocele: A multivariate statistical analysis. Samuelsson L, Skoog M. *J Pediatr Orthop* 1988;8:569-575.

One hundred sixty-three patients with myelomeningocele were studied by multivariate statistical analysis. No ambulators were found at the thoracic or L1-L2 levels. Below L1-L2, one half of the non-ambulators had neurologic deficiencies such as syringohydromyelia or Chiari malformation demonstrated on magnetic resonance imaging. In the other non-ambulators, severe scoliosis was closely, age was moderately, and hip flexion contracture was slightly related to the inability to walk.

211

Significance of the strength of the quadriceps muscles in children with myelomeningocele. Schopler SA, Menelaus MB. *J Pediatr Orthop* 1987;7:507-512.

> One hundred nine patients with myelomeningocele were assessed at an average age of 12.5 years (range 6 to 26 years). Eighty-nine percent with grade 3, 4, or 5 quadriceps power were at least household ambulators. Conversely, 88% of patients with grade 0, 1, or 2 quadriceps strength were exclusively wheelchair users. Quadriceps power can be assessed in the first 3 years of life. Those children who have a grade 4 or 5 quadriceps power in the first 3 years have a high probability of unchanged or improved knee extensor strength, whereas those with a quadriceps power of grade 2 or less have a high probability of persisting in this state.

Orthopaedic management of high-level spina bifida: Early walking compared with early use of a wheelchair. Mazur JM, Shurtleff D, Menelaus M, et al. *J Bone Joint Surg* 1989;71A:56-61.

> Two groups of high level myelomeningocele children, controlled for age, sex, level of lesion, and intelligence, were compared. Group I had participated in a walking program; group II had a wheelchair prescribed early in life. Group I had fewer fractures and pressure sores, were more independent, and were better able to do independent wheelchair transfers. Group II had spent fewer days in the hospital. No major differences were found between the groups with regard to skills of daily living, hand function, or obesity.

Bone density in myelomeningocele: The effects of ambulatory status and other factors. Rosenstein BD, Greene WB, Herrington RT, et al. *Dev Med Child Neurol* 1987;29:486-494.

> Multivariate analysis was made of single photon bone density measurements of the distal radius, mid-radius, tibia, and first metatarsal in 80 patients with myelomeningocele. Upper-extremity measurements were decreased only in the thoracic level patients. Lower-extremity bone strength had a more linear correlation with neurologic level. Patients with impaired ambulation had decreased bone density in the distal radius, tibia, and metatarsal, but not in the mid-radius. Neurologic status seemed to be more important than level of ambulatory function in determining bone density.

Spine

Osteotomy-excision of the spine for lumbar kyphosis in older children with myelomeningocele. Sharrard WJW, Drennan JC. *J Bone Joint Surg* 1972;54B:50-60.

> The etiology, anatomy, and prognosis in untreated cases of lumbar kyphosis in myelomeningocele is reviewed. The authors describe a technique of osteotomy-vertebral body excision. The level of osteotomy depends on whether the compensatory thoracic lordosis is supple or

fixed. Describes results in 14 children who had the procedure at an older age and in 13 children who had the procedure as a newborn.

Vertebral excision for kyphosis in children with myelomeningocele. Lindseth RE, Stelzer L Jr. *J Bone Joint Surg* 1979;61A:699-704.

Twenty-three children with myelomeningocele underwent 3 types of operations, all including vertebral excision. Partial resection of the apical vertebrae and of the proximal lordotic curve provided more persistent correction than did wedge excision based on the apical vertebrae.

Excision and wire fixation of rigid myelomeningocele kyphosis. Christofersen MR, Brooks AL. *J Pediatr Orthop* 1985:691-696.

Results of vertebral excision and wire fixation in 9 children with myelomeningocele are described. Mean follow-up was 5.4 years. Complications were frequent but the goals of postural stability and skin ulceration control were achieved. Significant loss of correction obtained at surgery was frequent.

Management of myelomeningocele kyphosis in the older child by kyphectomy and segmental spinal instrumentation. Heydemann JS, Gillespie R. *Spine* 1987;12:37-41.

Twelve patients with myelomeningocele kyphosis measuring an average of 124 degrees were managed by posterior kyphectomy and segmental spinal instrumentation with anterior fixation to the pelvis. After operation, the curves measured an average of 33 degrees. Only one patient lost correction in the follow-up period ranging from six to 57 months.

The long-term results of kyphectomy and spinal stabilization in children with myelomeningocele. McMaster MJ. *Spine* 1988;13:417-424.

Ten patients with severe lumbar kyphosis were treated by resection of the kyphus, internal fixation, and spine fusion. The authors note that this major procedure was associated with many complications including one death. The nine patients followed to skeletal maturity had a flat back without pressure sores and were able to sit upright without using their arms for support.

Paralytic spinal deformity: Orthotic treatment in spinal discontinuity syndromes. Johnston CE II, Hakala MW, Rosenberger R. *J Pediatr Orthop* 1982;2:233-244.

Treatment with total contact orthoses to postpone spinal stabilization in 19 children with paralytic spinal deformity was reviewed. Average time of brace treatment was 54 months. The curvatures averaged 43 degrees prior to treatment, 26 degrees at best correction, and 39 degrees at last follow-up or when the brace was discontinued. Unacceptable progression was associated with poor compliance.

Surgical treatment of paralytic scoliosis associated with myelomeningocele. Osebold WR, Mayfield JK, Winter RB, et al. *J Bone Joint Surg* 1982;64A:841-856.

> The combination of anterior and posterior fusion with instrumentation was significantly better compared with posterior fusion and instrumentation alone in 40 patients with myelomeningocele and paralytic scoliosis. Fusion across the lumbosacral joint even with Harrington rods was a persistent problem.

Improvement in pulmonary function in patients having combined anterior and posterior spine fusion for myelomeningocele scoliosis. Banta JV, Park SM. *Spine* 1983;8:765-770.

> In ten myelomeningocele patients having anterior and posterior spine fusion, vital capacity was not altered. When the scoliosis was greater than 60 degrees, fusion improved measurements of pulmonary mechanics, such as peak flow and maximum voluntary ventilation.

Surgical correction of myelomeningocele scoliosis: A critical appraisal of various spinal instrumentation systems. Ward WT, Wenger DR, Roach JW. *J Pediatr Orthop* 1989;9:262-268.

> Thirty-eight patients with myelomeningocele scoliosis were reviewed. Single stage anterior or posterior procedures resulted in a 50% fusion rate compared to rates of 83 to 100% for various combinations of combined anterior and posterior fusions. Average curve correction and change in pelvic obliquity were also much improved with the two-stage approach. No statistical difference in fusion rate, curve correction, or change in pelvic obliquity was found between the various combinations of two-stage operations.

Efficacy of surgical management for scoliosis in myelomeningocele: Correction of deformity and alteration of functional status. Mazur J, Menelaus MB, Dickens DR, et al. *J Pediatr Orthop* 1986;6:568-575.

> In 49 patients with myelomeningocele undergoing spine fusion for scoliosis, the authors found that sitting was likely to be improved, but ambulation might be adversely affected. Patients and their parents should be aware of this potential change.

MR imaging of syringohydromyelia and Chiari malformations in myelomeningocele patients with scoliosis. Samuelsson L, Bergström K, Thuomas KA, et al. *AJNR* 1987;8:539-546.

> The brain and spinal cord were examined with magnetic resonance imaging in 30 myelomeningocele patients. All patients had Chiari malformations, 28 of type II and 2 of type I. Syringohydromyelia was seen in 12 patients but was not correlated with the pattern of spinal curvature, result of ventricular shunt, level of myelomeningocele, or extent of the Chiari malformation. Rapid progression of scoliosis was associated with extensive syringohydromyelia.

Hip

The hip in myelomeningocele: Management directed towards a minimum number of operations and a minimum period of immobilisation. Menelaus MB. *J Bone Joint Surg* 1976;58B:448-452.

> The author reviews his experience with 116 myelomeningocele children. Children who lack strong quadriceps muscles are treated by simple procedures, such as tendon releases to correct contractures. Tendon transfers and bony reconstructions are reserved for patients with a strong quadriceps muscle. Principles of management outlined by the author should be understood by all orthopaedic surgeons who take care of children with myelomeningocele.

Posterior iliopsoas transplantation in the treatment of paralytic dislocation of the hip. Sharrard WJW. *J Bone Joint Surg* 1964;46B:426-444.

> A classic.

Long-term follow-up of posterior iliopsoas transplantation for paralytic dislocation of the hip. Carroll NC, Sharrard WJW. *J Bone Joint Surg* 1972;54A:551-560.

> Thirty-three children (58 hips) were reviewed after posterior iliopsoas transplantation. Of these patients, 70% underwent additional or concomitant femoral osteotomies and adductor tenotomies. Instability, still present in 40%, was most commonly caused by failure to achieve a stable concentric reduction at the time of surgery. Based on this study, the authors recommend simpler soft-tissue releases for the child with a high level paraplegia.

Factors affecting the ambulatory status of patients with spina bifida cystica. Asher M, Olson J. *J Bone Joint Surg* 1983;65A:350-356.

> Hip deformity was found to be a significant variable affecting ambulatory status in the L3-L4 level myelomeningocele patient, but was not significant in the thoracic or L1-L2 group. The authors recommend that with L4 level myelomeningocele, unilateral or bilateral dislocation should be prevented if possible, or treated if present. For thoracic or L1-L2 myelomeningocele, hip dislocation should be ignored and contractures released as necessary. For patients with L3 level myelomeningocele, the authors favored treatment for a unilateral dislocation and simple release of contractures for bilateral dislocation unless there was a reliable method of maintaining reduction.

Hip stability and ambulatory status in myelomeningocele. Lee EH, Carroll NC. *J Pediatr Orthop* 1985;5:522-527.

> Fifty-three hips in patients with myelomeningocele and innervation to the quadriceps were surgically stabilized. Before surgery, 93% of the hips were either subluxated or dislocated. At review, 83% of the hips were stable.

Effectiveness of muscle transfers in myelomeningocele hips measured by radiographic indices. Yngve DA, Lindseth RE. *J Pediatr Orthop* 1982;2:121-125.

> Surgery (Sharrard transfer or external oblique transfer, with or without adductor release or adductor transfer) was evaluated in 35 hips in ambulatory myelomeningocele patients. In some patients, femoral osteotomy was performed. When abductor and adductor procedures were not combined, only 6 of 26 hips were improved radiographically. The authors presently favor the external oblique transfer over the iliopsoas transfer.

Abduction splinting of the hip joints in myelodysplastic infants. Raycroft JF. *J Pediatr Orthop* 1987;7:686-689.

> To prevent secondary adaptive acetabular changes and decrease the number and complexity of hip reconstructive procedures, patients with mid-lumbar level myelomeningocele were treated with abduction hip splinting until age 2. An unsplinted control group had poor results. The splinted group had better hip stability and a decreased frequency of femoral and pelvic osteotomies.

Knee and Lower Limb

Surgical management of knee contractures in myelomeningocele. Dias LS. *J Pediatr Orthop* 1982;2:127-131.

> In 23 knees a radical flexor release demonstrated post-operative contractures of 10 degrees or less in 91%. A simple tendon release in 3 knees produced a poor result. Fifteen knees had successful treatment of extension contracture by a VY quadriceps lengthening.

Knee flexion contractures in myelodysplasia. Nunley JA, Sperduto PW. *South Med J* 1986;79:818-821.

> Twenty-one knees were treated by either femoral osteotomy alone or soft-tissue lengthening of the hamstring tendons and release of the posterior capsule with or without femoral osteotomy. The group treated by femoral osteotomy alone produced 40% unsatisfactory results.

Rotational deformities of the lower limb in myelomeningocele: evaluation and treatment. Dias LS, Jasty MJ, Collins P. *J Bone Joint Surg* 1984;66A:215-223.

> Surgical treatment and its results were described for rotational deformities in 50 myelomeningocele children. Rotational deformities were classified as (1) external rotation deformity of the hip, (2) external tibial torsion, and (3) toeing in gait either secondary to medial-lateral hamstring imbalance, to internal tibial torsion, or to a combination of muscle imbalance and bony deformity.

Ankle and Foot

Management of the foot in spinal dysraphism and myelodysplasias. Duckworth T. In Jahss MH (ed): *Disorders of the Foot.* Philadelphia, WB Saunders, 1982, vol 1, pp. 248-281.
> A comprehensive discussion of pathogenesis, assessment, principles of treatment, and management of specific deformities.

Valgus deformity of the ankle in myelodysplastic patients: Correction by stapling of the medial part of the distal tibial physis. Burkus JK, Moore DW, Raycroft JF. *J Bone Joint Surg* 1983;65A:1157-1162.
> Stapling of the distal medial tibial physis for a valgus deformity of the ankle was evaluated in 12 myelomeningocele patients. Average correction was 16 degrees, and there were no major complications. The method was recommended as safe, simple, and effective.

The results of transfer of the tibialis anterior to the heel in patients who have a myelomeningocele. Bliss DG, Menelaus MB. *J Bone Joint Surg* 1986;68A:1258-1264.
> Forty-six transfers of the tibialis anterior to the os calcis were reviewed. Patients operated on after the age of 5 years had better results. Equinus developed in 14 feet, and 8 of these required release of the transferred tendon. The authors thought that these patients had unrecognized spasticity in the transferred muscles.

Anterior tibial transfer to the os calcis with Achilles tenodesis for calcaneal deformity in myelomeningocele. Banta JV, Sutherland DH, Wyatt M. *J Pediatr Orthop* 1981;1:125-130.
> Seven children who underwent transfer of the anterior tibial muscle to the os calcis combined with Achilles tenodesis were analyzed by pre- and post-operative gait studies. Decreased knee flexion and ankle dorsiflexion in stance were found. Work output was lessened. Post-operative orthotic support was important for long-term function.

Correction of combined tibial torsion and valgus deformity of the foot. Nicol RO, Menelaus MB. *J Bone Joint Surg* 1983;65B:641-645.
> A supramalleolar tibial osteotomy combined with a lateral inlay triple arthrodesis was performed on 20 feet and reviewed after an average follow-up of three years. The combination of deformities was fully corrected in 75%, and the use of calipers was minimized in 95%. Complications included recurrent valgus deformity, delayed union of the tibial osteotomy, and failure of mid-tarsal fusion.

Talectomy in the treatment of resistant talipes equinovarus deformity in myelomeningocele and arthrogryposis. Dias LS, Stern LS. *J Pediatr Orthop* 1987;7:39-41.
> Twenty-eight feet in patients with spina bifida and arthrogryposis underwent talectomy to correct severe equinovarus deformity. A

posterior medial release had been performed previously in 26 feet. Six feet required metatarsal osteotomy to correct forefoot adduction.

Ground-reaction forces on the plantar surface of the foot after talectomy in the myelomeningocele. Sherk HH, Marchinski LJ, Clancy M, et al. *J Pediatr Orthop* 1989;9:269-275.
> Force-plate analysis was done on 19 patients at 12.6 years after talectomy. An apparently plantigrade foot was usually obtained, but talectomy rarely succeeded in distributing weightbearing forces uniformly over the plantar surface.

Subtalar arthrodesis in children. Gallien R, Morin F, Marquis F. *J Pediatr Orthop* 1989;9:59-63.
> Subtalar arthrodesis had a larger percentage of unsatisfactory results (39%) in children with myelomeningocele. Residual valgus related to deformity in the ankle and forepart of the foot was the most frequent problem.

Orthoses

Comparison of plastic/metal and leather/metal knee ankle-foot orthoses. Krebs DE, Edelstein JE, Fishman S. *Am J Phys Med Rehabil* 1988;67:175-185.
> Fifteen children had alternate fitting of plastic/metal and leather/metal long leg braces. Although no overall functional differences were found between the two types, most children preferred the plastic/metal orthoses since they were lighter and more easily donned and doffed. The plastic/metal orthoses also more effectively controlled hip and knee sagittal motion and foot valgus/varus position during gait.

A clinical review of the orthotic treatment of myelomeningocele patients. Rose GK, Sankarankutty M, Stallard J. *J Bone Joint Surg* 1983;65B:242-246.
> The authors describe a swivel walker and hip guidance orthosis for patients with high myelomeningocele lesions. With these orthoses, a higher percentage of patients achieved functional ambulation.

Ambulation of children with myelomeningocele: Parapodium versus parapodium with Orlau swivel modification. Lough LK, Nielsen DH. *Dev Med Child Neurol* 1986;28:489-497.
> Ten paraplegic children were analyzed using two orthotic devices. Walking velocities were significantly higher with the parapodium, but energy costs and gait efficiency were significantly better with the swivel walker.

The reciprocating gait orthosis in myelomeningocele. Yngve DA, Douglas R, Roberts JM. *J Pediatr Orthop* 1984;4:304-310.
> Seventeen patients with myelomeningocele were fitted with a device that reciprocally controlled hip flexion and extension. The orthosis was most successful when strong hip flexors were present.

Polypropylene lower-extremity braces for paraplegia due to myelomeningocele. Lindseth RE, Glancy J. *J Bone Joint Surg* 1974;56A:556-563.

> A polypropylene ankle-foot orthosis with an anterior proximal tibial shell was applied to 47 children with an L3-L5 level myelomeningocele. Bracing requirements (compared with previously used conventional double upright, metal braces) were reduced in 18 patients.

Inflammatory Conditions

G. Paul DeRosa, MD

Juvenile Rheumatoid Arthritis

Chronic arthritis in children: Juvenile rheumatoid arthritis. Schaller JG. *Clin Orthop* 1984;182:79-89.
> Juvenile rheumatoid arthritis, best defined as the condition of chronic synovitis in children, probably includes several distinct disease processes. There are no diagnostic laboratory tests, and various subgroups differ in immunogenetic findings as well as in clinical appearance and prognosis. A wide variety of conditions that mimic JRA must be considered in the diagnosis.

The management of chronic arthritis of children. Ansell BM, Swann M. *J Bone Joint Surg* 1983;65B:536-543.
> Conservative and surgical treatment of JRA are discussed with emphasis on the special problems of children with arthritis. Early diagnosis and proper treatment are the keys to successful management.

Monarticular juvenile rheumatoid arthritis. Blockey NJ, Gibson AA, Goel KM. *J Bone Joint Surg* 1980;62B:368-371.
> Seven of 22 children with monarticular juvenile rheumatoid arthritis developed involvement of other joints between 6 months and 3.5 years after onset. In the other 15, the disease remained monarticular for between 1 and 16 years (mean 6 years). Children with monarticular juvenile rheumatoid arthritis and antinuclear antibodies should have periodic ophthalmic assessment to rule out chronic iridocyclitis. Synovial biopsy was of value primarily in excluding other causes of arthritis.

MR imaging in juvenile rheumatoid arthritis. Senac MO Jr, Deutsch D, Bernstein BH, et al. *AJR* 1988;150:873-878.
> Twenty-one patients with juvenile rheumatoid arthritis and three normal volunteers were studied with magnetic resonance scanner. Cartilage space narrowing, popliteal cysts, and fluid within the joints were shown with greater accuracy than on conventional radiography.

Late results of synovectomy in juvenile rheumatoid arthritis. Jacobsen ST, Levinson JE, Crawford AH. *J Bone Joint Surg* 1985;67A:8-15.
> There were few if any benefits from the operation with reference to pain or improvement of range of motion. The authors have not done the

procedure since 1978 but state that there may still be an indication for the operation in certain patients with long-standing pauciarticular synovitis.

Comparison of synovectomy and no synovectomy in patients with juvenile rheumatoid arthritis: A 24-month controlled study. Kvien TK, Pahle JA, Høyeraal HM, et al. *Scand J Rheumatol* 1987;16:81-91.
> Efficacy of synovectomy was evaluated in 30 patients with juvenile rheumatoid arthritis. Patients were randomly assigned to receive or not receive synovectomy. At the end of the study, no active disease was detected in 8 of the 15 patients who had synovectomy, whereas all joints in the non-synovectomized group had active disease. The synovectomy group lost motion compared to the non-operated group.

Changes in the cervical spine in juvenile rheumatoid arthritis. Hensinger RN, DeVito PD, Ragsdale CG. *J Bone Joint Surg* 1986;68A:189-198.
> The authors studied 121 patients with juvenile rheumatoid arthritis for disease of the cervical spine. Of 57 patients with pauciarticular onset, none had cervical signs or symptoms and only one had radiographic changes. In 51 patients with polyarticular onset and in 13 patients with systemic onset, clinical stiffness and radiographic changes occurred. Authors conclude that severe pain in the neck and torticollis should be investigated for an intercurrent problem, such as fracture or infection, because severe pain is rarely secondary to rheumatoid arthritis.

The cervical spine in juvenile rheumatoid arthritis. Fried JA, Athreya B, Gregg JR, et al. *Clin Orthop* 1983;179:102-106.
> Clinical and roentgenographic follow-up examination of patients with juvenile rheumatoid arthritis suggest that neurologic complications are less likely to develop in these patients than in patients with adult rheumatoid arthritis.

The hand in the child with juvenile rheumatoid arthritis. Granberry WM, Mangum GL. *J Hand Surg* 1980;5:105-113.
> Clinical examination of 100 children showed frequent ulnar deviation and loss of wrist extension. Loss of flexion and radial deviation in the metacarpophalangeal joint is more frequent than in the adult. Statistical review of charts and radiographs of 200 patients showed all had ulnar shortening (up to 9 mm), but there was no correlation with ulnar deviation or metacarpophalangeal radial deviation. Conservative treatment is recommended; surgery is rarely indicated.

Involvement of the hip in juvenile rheumatoid arthritis: A longitudinal study. Harris CM, Baum J. *J Bone Joint Surg* 1988;70A:821-833.
> Thirty-five children with rheumatoid arthritis were followed for up to 22 years. Four categories of involvement were seen. Group I, mild disability, minimal changes radiographically. Group II, two patients with episodic disability. Group III, 14 patients with progressive disability and radiographic changes. Of 59 operations, 55 were performed on children of group III. Group IV, 6 patients with

significant clinical and radiographic findings, but with little functional disability at time of follow-up.

Arthroscopy of the hip in juvenile chronic arthritis. Holgersson S, Brattström H, Mogensen B, et al. *J Pediatr Orthop* 1981;1:273-278.

Hip arthroscopy performed in 13 patients (15 hips) with juvenile chronic arthritis gave better information about the cartilage than did roentgenograms and gave the same information about the synovial membrane as did an open operation. This diagnostic method is recommended early in the course of hip disability.

Femoral head necrosis in juvenile chronic arthritis. Kobayakawa M, Rydholm U, Wingstrand H, et al. *Acta Orthop Scand* 1989;60:164-169.

Of 206 children with juvenile chronic arthritis, 36 presented with hip pain or limited motion. Of ten hips with obvious signs of femoral head necrosis, nine showed a sclerotic rim at the base of the femoral neck, which was interpreted as evidence of earlier ischemic damage to the epiphysis and growth plate. The authors conclude that femoral head necrosis in juvenile rheumatoid arthritis is more common than previously reported and may be caused by circulatory disturbances secondary to increased intra-articular pressure caused by synovitis and/or effusion.

Synovectomy of the hip in juvenile chronic arthritis. Mogensen B, Brattström H, Ekelund L, et al. *J Bone Joint Surg* 1982;64B:295-299.

Eighteen synovectomies of the hip in 16 patients with juvenile chronic arthritis were performed with satisfactory relief of pain in 13 hips. The average age of the patients was 14 years with a follow-up of 52 months. Mobility and walking capacity were not changed. Synovectomy may relieve pain permanently and should be considered before prosthetic replacement.

Total hip replacement in juvenile chronic arthritis. Mogensen B, Brattström H, Ekelund L, et al. *Acta Orthop Scand* 1983;54:422-430.

Long-term follow-up (average 6.5 years) of 50 total hip replacements in 33 patients with juvenile rheumatoid arthritis (41 hips) and ankylosing spondylitis (9 hips) showed satisfactory results concerning pain relief, increased range of hip motion, and decreased flexion contractures. Twelve percent required further surgery because of infection or loosening. The authors recommend delaying joint replacement for the young patient as long as possible and suggest the use of arthroscopy of the hip to assess the status of the cartilage.

Total hip and total knee arthroplasty in juvenile rheumatoid arthritis. Scott RD, Sarokhan AJ, Dalziel R. *Clin Orthop* 1984;182:90-98.

Total hip or total knee arthroplasty is indicated for patients with juvenile rheumatoid arthritis when marked joint destruction is present and pain or deformity compromises function despite optimal medical therapy. Relief of pain, reduction of the deformity, and dramatic improvement in functional status and quality of life can be achieved in most patients.

Severe generalized (Charcot-like) joint destruction in juvenile rheumatoid arthritis. Rothschild BM, Hanissian AS. *Clin Orthop* 1981;155:75-80.

> Histopathologic examination of two children with severe polyarticular joint destruction associated with juvenile rheumatoid arthritis revealed fragments of cartilage imbedded in synovial membrane, such as are usually seen in adults with neuropathic joint disease. Steroid hormone treatment may be implicated in pathogenesis of joint destruction in children.

Juvenile psoriatic arthritis: An analysis of 60 cases. Shore A, Ansell BM. *J Pediatr* 1982;100:529-535.

> Of 60 children with juvenile psoriatic arthritis, the majority had a monarticular presentation, usually of the knee. Additional joints usually became involved sporadically in an asymmetric pattern, in both the upper and lower extremity, so that 87% ultimately had polyarticular disease. Although 40% were asymptomatic at follow-up, six required bilateral hip replacement within five years following onset of arthritis.

Seronegative Spondyloarthropathies

The seronegative spondyloarthropathies of childhood. Schaller JG. *Clin Orthop* 1979;143:76-83.

> Most chronic arthritis in children is seronegative. Of the several distinct subgroups of juvenile rheumatoid arthritis, recognition of patients with pauciarticular disease type II is important to permit proper therapy, follow-up, and prevention of deformity.

Ankylosing spondylitis and its variants: A review of recent developments for orthopaedic surgeons. Cheatum DE, Kier CM. *Clin Orthop* 1977;129:196-200.

> Ankylosing spondylitis has been shown to be separate and distinct from rheumatoid arthritis. The HL-A B27 genetic test is used to identify ankylosing spondylitis patients, and radioisotopic bone and joint scanning augment diagnosis. Inappropriate treatment or procedures can be avoided by proper diagnosis.

Nonsteroidal anti-inflammatory agents in rheumatoid arthritis and ankylosing spondylitis. Wasner C, Britton MC, Kraines RG, et al. *JAMA* 1981;246:2168-2172.

> A study of the relative effectiveness of six nonsteroidal anti-inflammatory agents in 33 patients with rheumatoid arthritis and 32 patients with ankylosing spondylitis showed naproxen, indomethacin, and fenoprofen the most effective agents in ankylosing spondylitis. In rheumatoid arthritis, relatively little mean difference between drugs was found.

Therapy of the spondyloarthropathies. Smythe H. *Clin Orthop* 1979;143:84-89.

The recommended treatment for patients with ankylosing spondylitis is a life-long exercise program, frequently with concomitant nonsteroidal anti-inflammatory drug therapy. This therapeutic program ensures good functional prognosis in the vast majority of patients.

Nonreducible rotational head tilt and atlantoaxial lateral mass collapse: Clinical and roentgenographic features in patients with juvenile rheumatoid arthritis and ankylosing spondylitis. Halla JT, Fallahi S, Hardin JG. *Arch Intern Med* 1983;143:471-474.

Nonreducible rotational head tilt resulting from predominantly unilateral collapse of the lateral mass of the atlas and/or axis was found in five patients with juvenile rheumatoid arthritis and six with ankylosing spondylitis. Most patients had neck pain and crepitus, all had a fixed head tilt deformity, and most also had a rotational deformity. Patients with ankylosing spondylitis tended to have more severe neck symptoms and to require surgery more often than those with juvenile rheumatoid arthritis.

Spontaneous atlantoaxial subluxation as a presenting manifestation of juvenile ankylosing spondylitis: A case report. Thompson GH, Khan MA, Bilenker RM. *Spine* 1982;7:78-79.

Atlantoaxial instability and neck pain without neurologic involvement were presenting manifestations of juvenile ankylosing spondylitis in one patient. Laboratory and clinical features of juvenile ankylosing spondylitis are discussed, along with the importance of qualitative sacroiliac joint scintigraphy in the diagnosis of early or confusing cases.

Seronegative inflammations of the ankle and foot: Diagnostic challenges. Capen D, Scheck M. *Clin Orthop* 1981;155:147-155.

Seronegative inflammatory disease was diagnosed in seven patients who had pain, swelling, and redness of the foot and/or ankle. Clinical findings mimicked infection, tendinitis, fasciitis, or chronic strain. HLA-B27 antigen, technetium-99m diphosphonate scintigraphy, and magnification roentgenograms have proven useful in diagnosing seronegative inflammatory disease.

Hemophilia and Other Hematologic Disorders

Walter B. Greene, MD

Hemophilia

Hemophilic arthropathy: Current concepts of pathogenesis and management.
Arnold WD, Hilgartner MW. *J Bone Joint Surg* 1977;59A:287-305.
> This landmark article discusses the clinical presentation,
> pathophysiology, and treatment of hemophilic arthropathy and soft
> tissue bleeds.

The pathogenesis of chronic haemophilic arthropathy. Stein H, Duthie RB. *J
Bone Joint Surg* 1981;63B:601-609.
> Specimens of tissue from hemophilic synovium and articular cartilage
> were collected from 39 patients. Findings suggest that hemophilic
> arthropathy results from mechanisms affecting the synovial lining,
> which becomes progressively fibrotic, and the hyaline cartilage, which
> disintegrates and is eventually lost.

Mechanisms of joint damage in an experimental model of hemophilic arthritis.
Madhok R, Bennett D, Sturrock RD, et al. *Arthritis Rheum* 1988;31:1148-
1155.
> Autologous whole blood was injected the knee joints of rabbits 3 times
> each week for 12 weeks. Immunofluorescence studies indicated that a
> specific immune response is probably not involved in the pathogenesis
> of hemophilic arthritis. Detailed histopathologic examination revealed an
> obvious iron overload in the synovium and cartilage.

Nonsurgical management of hemophilic arthropathy. Greene WB, McMillan
CW. In Barr JS Jr (ed): American Academy of Orthopaedic Surgeons
Instructional Course Lectures XXXVIII. Park Ridge, IL, American Academy
of Orthopaedic Surgeons, 1989, pp 367-381.
> This article reviews normal clotting mechanisms and the deficiencies in
> the coagulation disorders. Discusses the pathogenesis, radiographic
> evaluation, and nonsurgical management of hemophilic arthropathy.

Clinical features of early haemarthroses in severely affected adolescent
haemophiliacs. Aronstam A, Browne RS, Wassef M, et al. *Clin Lab Haematol*
1984;6:9-15.
> Studies 690 bleeds into the knees, ankles, and elbows of severe
> hemophiliacs who were treated within three hours of the onset of

symptoms. Stiffness, pain, and tenderness were common complaints. There was a direct relationship between the degree of swelling, extent of movement restriction, and time taken for complete restoration of function, the mean of which was 3.6 days for elbows, 2.5 for knees, and 1.1 for ankles.

Five stages of joint disintegration compared with range of motion in hemophilia. Johnson RP, Babbitt DP. *Clin Orthop* 1985;201:36-42.
A roentgenographic classification system was compared to the arc of motion for the knee, elbow, and ankle in patients with severe hemophilia. With advancing arthropathy, the mean arc of motion demonstrated a progressive decrease that was quantified for each joint. Lack of elbow extension, knee flexion, and ankle dorsiflexion characterize the early stages of arthropathy.

Roentgenographic classifications of hemophilic arthropathy: Comparison of three systems and correlation with clinical parameters. Greene WB, Yankaskas BC, Guilford WB. *J Bone Joint Surg* 1989;71A:237-244.
In 105 knees, two commonly used roentgenographic classifications of hemophilic arthropathy and a new system were compared. The system of Pettersson and associates was better than that of Arnold and Hilgartner for grading severe arthropathy, but it was not better than the new, simplified system. The new system is a four-sign, 7-point classification in contrast to the eight-sign, 13-point Pettersson system.

Surgical management of hemophilic arthropathy. DeGnore LT, Wilson FC. In Barr JS Jr (ed): American Academy of Orthopaedic Surgeons *Instructional Course Lectures, XXXVIII*. Park Ridge, IL, American Academy Of Orthopaedic Surgeons, 1989, pp 383-388.
This article reviews the hematologic management of patients with hemophilia undergoing surgery. The results of surgery are also discussed.

Synovectomy of the knee for hemophilic arthropathy. Montane I, McCollough NC III, Lian EC. *J Bone Joint Surg* 1986;68A:210-216.
Synovectomy of the knee for the control of recurrent hemarthrosis was performed in 13 patients. Ten patients lost an average of 41 degrees of knee motion, but the incidence of hemarthrosis was markedly decreased. This procedure also appeared to slow the progression of the arthropathy.

Synovectomy of the knee in hemophilia. Nicol RO, Menelaus MB. *J Pediatr Orthop* 1986;6:330-333.
Ten children underwent synovectomy of the knee with marked reduction in the frequency and severity of bleeding. Continuous passive motion was important in postoperative management, but joint manipulation was of doubtful value.

Synoviorthesis with colloidal 32P chromic phosphate for hemophilic arthropathy: Clinical follow-up. Rivard GE, Girard M, Lamarre C, et al. *Arch Phys Med Rehabil* 1985;66:753-756.

> Thirty-one synoviortheses were performed in 22 joints of 14 hemophilic patients. Frequency and severity of bleeding decreased in all patients. Results in patients with high titer factor VIII inhibitors were comparable to those in hemophiliacs without inhibitors.

Orthopaedic procedures and prognosis in hemophilic patients who are seropositive for human immunodeficiency virus. Greene WB, DeGnore LT, White GC. *J Bone Joint Surg* 1990;72A:2-11.

> The rate of nosocomial infection and the results of surgical therapy were not adversely affected in 30 hemophiliacs who were HIV seropositive; however, abnormal postoperative temperature elevation without the expected elevation in the white blood cell count was seen in five cases. The authors advocate preoperative assessment of immune competence by measuring the CD4 lymphocyte count and intradermal skin tests.

Acquired immune deficiency syndrome associated with hemophilia in the United States. Stehr-Green JK, Evatt BL, Lawrence DN. In Barr JS Jr (ed): American Academy of Orthopaedic Surgeons *Instructional Course Lectures, XXXVIII*. Park Ridge, IL, American Academy of Orthopaedic Surgeons, 1989, pp 357-365.

> The anthors, who are physicians at the Centers for Disease Control, review the etiology, incidence, and risk of HIV transmission in hemophiliacs. Guidelines for healthcare professionals are discussed.

HIV and hemophilic children's growth. Jason J, Gomperts E, Lawrence DN, et al. *J Acquir Immune Defic Syndr* 1989;2:277-282.

> The effect of the human immunodeficiency virus was studied in four groups of hemophilic children.

Hemoglobinopathies

Bone and joint lesions in sickle-cell disease. Diggs LW. *Clin Orthop* 1967;52:119-143.

> A classic.

Osteomyelitis in the patient with sickle-cell disease: Diagnosis and management. Engh CA, Hughes JL, Abrams RC, et al. *J Bone Joint Surg* 1971;53A:1-15.

> Salmonella bone infections, although rare in the overall population, occur frequently in patients with sickle-cell disease. Early diagnosis is imperative; delayed or inadequate antibiotic therapy can be disastrous. Clinical symptoms include persistent spiking fever, persistent leukocytosis, and roentgenographic changes far more dramatic than those secondary to thrombotic bone crises.

Etiology of osteomyelitis in patients with major sickle hemoglobinopathies. Givner LB, Luddy RE, Schwartz AD. *J Pediatr* 1981;99:411-413.

> A review of culture-proven reports of osteomyelitis in sickle cell anemia. In 84 patients, 68 (74%) were secondary to salmonella, whereas Staphylococcus accounted for only 10%.

Bone and joint infection in patients with sickle cell disease. Mallouh A, Talab Y. *J Pediatr Orthop* 1985;5:158-162.

> Twelve cases of bone and/or joint infection were reviewed in patients with sickle cell disease. Long bone and multiple site involvement were common. Differentiation from acute bony infarcts is difficult, and a systemic and aggressive approach to early diagnosis, management, and follow-up is suggested.

Osteomyelitis and infarction in sickle cell hemoglobinopathies: Differentiation by combined technetium and gallium scintigraphy. Amundsen TR, Siegel MJ, Siegel BA. *Radiology* 1984;153:807-812.

> Eighteen patients had combined scans during 22 separate episodes of suspected osseous infection. Overall, the results indicate that the combination of technetium and gallium scintigraphy is an effective means to distinguish osteomyelitis from infarction in patients with sickle cell hemoglobinopathies.

Scintigraphic differentiation of bone infarction from osteomyelitis in children with sickle cell disease. Rao S, Solomon N, Miller S, et al. *J Pediatr* 1985;107:685-688.

> Bone scans, bone marrow scans, or both were obtained during 42 episodes of bone pain in 40 children with sickle cell disease. Bone marrow scans were more useful than bone scans for differentiating infarction from osteomyelitis.

Pathological fracture complicating long bone osteomyelitis in patients with sickle cell disease. Ebong, WW. *J Pediatr Orthop* 1986;6:177-181.

> In 266 consecutive major skeletal complications seen in patients with sickle cell disease, the following were encountered: osteomyelitis, 40.5%; aseptic necrosis of the femoral head, 28.2%; septic arthritis, 11.7%; pathologic fracture complicating long bone osteomyelitis, 9.8%; and miscellaneous complications, 1.8%. Pathologic fracture of long bones complicated osteomyelitis in 26 of 129 patients. The fracture was significantly more common in acute than in chronic osteomyelitis and in gram negative than in Staphylococcal infection. In these patients, the affected extremities should be adequately immobilized.

Observations on the natural history of dactylitis in homozygous sickle cell disease. Stevens MC, Padwick M, Serjeant GR. *Clin Pediatr (Phila)* 1981;20:311-317.

> In a prospective study, the authors evaluated dactylitis or hand-foot syndrome. The overall incidence was 45%. Of the affected patients, 41% demonstrated recurrent episodes up to 4 years of age. The problem

was not seen after 6 years of age--the cessation of dactylitis coincided with the disappearance of hematopoietic marrow in the hands and feet.

Salmonella osteomyelitis and hand-foot syndrome in a child with sickle cell anemia. Greene WB, McMillan CW. *J Pediatr Orthop* 1987;7:716-718.
   The diagnostic dilemmas and appropriate screening studies for the child with sickle cell anemia and atypical hand-foot syndrome are described.

Necrosis of the femoral head associated with sickle-cell anemia and its genetic variants: A review of the literature and study of thirteen cases. Chung SMK, Ralston EL. *J Bone Joint Surg* 1969;51A:33-58.
   The authors describe three clinical and roentgenographic groups in sickle cell patients with hip disease. Group I has Perthes-like involvement and may obtain satisfactory result with protected weightbearing. Group II has localized involvement similar to osteochondritis dissecans. Group III has typical destructive changes of osteonecrosis. The study also noted necrosis of other bones besides the hip joint.

Avascular necrosis of the hip in the sickle cell hemoglobinopathies. Sebes JI, Kraus AP. *J Can Assoc Radiol* 1983;34:136-139.
   Of 281 patients, 28% had avascular necrosis of the femoral head. The degree of anemia did not correlate well with symptoms. Thirteen patients with osteonecrosis of the hip underwent hip replacement and four developed prosthesis-related complications.

Osteonecrosis of the hip in the sickle-cell diseases: Treatment and complications. Hanker GJ, Amstutz HC. *J Bone Joint Surg* 1988;70A:499-506.
   Results were not very satisfactory in 11 patients with sickle cell anemia who had an operation on the hip. Five of eight arthroplasties required early revision or excision. Perioperative blood loss was excessive and hospitalization was prolonged.

Total hip arthroplasty in patients who have sickle-cell hemoglobinopathy. Bishop AR, Roberson JR, Eckman JR, et al. *J Bone Joint Surg* 1988;70A:853-855.
   Eleven patients with sickle cell hemoglobinopathy had a total hip arthroplasty for avascular necrosis of the hip. Four patients needed a revision and three required a resection arthroplasty. Four patients had a serious infection after surgery.

Anemias: Thalassemia

Fractures in thalassemia. Dines DM, Canale VC, Arnold WD. *J Bone Joint Surg* 1976;58A:662-666.
   Patients with homozygous beta-thalassemia often have pathologic fractures that are frequently multiple and usually involve the lower extremity. Delayed healing and resultant deformities are common.

Asymptomatic compression fractures of the spine and premature closure of the epiphyses of long bones also develop in these patients.

Fractures and epiphyseal deformities in beta-thalassemia. Exarchou E, Politou C, Vretou E, et al. *Clin Orthop* 1984;189:229-233.
Of 62 patients with beta-thalassemia (Cooley's anemia), 20 had sustained fractures, and of these,12 had recurrent or multiple fractures. Thirty of the 62 had deformed limbs as a result of epiphyseal abnormalities.

Fracture patterns in thalassemia. Finsterbush A, Farber I, Mogle P, et al. *Clin Orthop* 1985;192:132-136.
Of 61 patients with homozygous beta-thalassemia, 30 had fractures. An additional four patients suffered acute pain in the ankle and knee joints related to subchondral microfractures that were confirmed by scintigraphy. Only fractures of the femoral neck demonstrated delay in healing. The fracture pattern was either horizontal or slightly oblique and resembled the pathologic fractures in osteoporotic patients. Premature fusion of the epiphysis was noted in 12 patients, but was not thought to be a result of a pathologic fracture.

Aseptic necrosis of femoral head complicating thalassemia. Orzincolo C, Castaldi G, Scutellari PN, et al. *Skeletal Radiol* 1986;15:541-544.
Four patients with homozygous beta-thalassemia developed aseptic necrosis of the femoral head during childhood. Prolonged healing and residual deformity were characteristic.

Premature epiphyseal fusion and extramedullary hematopoiesis in thalassemia. Colavita N, Orazi C, Danza SM, et al. *Skeletal Radiol* 1987;16:533-538.
Premature growth plate arrest occurred in nine of 55 patients more than 10 years old. The proximal humerus was involved in all patients. This complication was associated with a delay in beginning transfusion therapy.

Leukemia

Orthopaedic manifestations of leukemia in children. Rogalsky RJ, Black GB, Reed MH. *J Bone Joint Surg* 1986;68A:494-501.
In 107 patients less than 18 years of age with leukemia, the presenting complaints were musculoskeletal in 20.6% and included pain in the extremities, back pain, osteomyelitis, septic arthritis, or fracture. Radiographic abnormalities, present in 44% at the time of diagnosis, included osteopenia, lytic lesions, metaphyseal bands, periosteal new bone, and sclerotic lesions.

Skeletal scintigraphy and radiography at onset of acute lymphocytic leukemia in children. Clausen N, Gøtze A Pedersen H, et al. *Med Pediatr Oncol* 1983;11:291-296.

Technetium 99m skeletal scintigraphy performed at the time of diagnosis was evaluated in 24 children with acute lymphocytic leukemia. Typical findings were localized intense uptake in one or several metaphyses and increased uptake in the diaphysis. The number of radiographic abnormalities was inversely correlated with age, whereas scintigraphic abnormalities correlated with age.

Absence of prognostic significance of skeletal involvement in acute lymphocytic leukemia and non-Hodgkin lymphoma in children. Appell RG, Bühler T, Willich E, et al. *Pediatr Radiol* 1985;15:245-248.
Seventy-two skeletal surveys performed at time of diagnosis in children with acute lymphocytic leukemia and malignant non-Hodgkin's lymphoma were correlated with the subsequent clinical course. There was no significant correlation between the extent of the skeletal involvement and the survival time.

Childhood acute lymphoblastic leukemia presenting as "cold" lesions on bone scan: A report of two cases. Caudle RJ, Crawford AH, Gelfand MJ, et al. *J Pediatr Orthop* 1987;7:93-95.
Two patients with leukemia who presented with refusal to walk demonstrated large "cold" spots on bone scans. A mild anemia suggested further diagnostic modalities.

A prospective analysis of the frequency, course, and possible prognostic significance of the joint manifestations of childhood leukemia. Costello PB, Brecher ML, Starr JI, et al. *J Rheumatol* 1983;10:753-757.
In a prospective study of 28 leukemic children, 14 had objective joint findings. These findings varied in severity, were most frequently present in the knee (86%), and were found most frequently only at disease onset (50%).

Gaucher's Disease

Skeletal manifestations and treatment of Gaucher's disease: Review of twenty cases. Amstutz HC, Carey EJ. *J Bone Joint Surg* 1966;48A:670-701.
The most frequent skeletal complaint was pain in the hip, knee, shoulder, or spine. Periosteal reaction may produce systemic signs mimicking infection. The femur is usually the first bone to show changes and is the most frequently involved. Reconstructive surgery may be of considerable benefit, but carries the risk of hemorrhage and infection.

Gaucher's disease. Lachiewicz PF. *Orthop Clin North Am* 1984;15:765-774.
This is a review of the classification, pathophysiology, and clinical manifestations of Gaucher's disease. The orthopaedic manifestations of the disease include bone pain syndromes, pathologic fractures, and avascular necrosis of the femoral head.

Skeletal complications of Gaucher disease. Stowens DW, Teitelbaum SL, Kahn AJ, et al. *Medicine (Baltimore)* 1985;64:310-322.

> In this review of 327 patients, the authors summarize the skeletal problems associated with Gaucher's disease. They emphasize the variability of the problems ranging from the patient's being asymptomatic to severe disability associated with osteopenia, osteonecrosis, and pathologic fractures. A possible explanation for the bone crisis that occurs in Gaucher's disease is discussed.

Evaluation of Gaucher disease using magnetic resonance imaging. Rosenthal DI, Scott JA, Barranger J, et al. *J Bone Joint Surg* 1986;68A:802-808.

> Magnetic resonance imaging was used to study skeletal involvement in 24 patients with Gaucher's disease. A non-homogeneous distribution of abnormal T1 and T2 signals replaced marrow. The epiphyses were generally spared. Proximal femoral areas were more frequently affected than distal tibial sites. Magnetic resonance imaging is more sensitive than computed tomography scanning.

Osteomyelitis in Gaucher disease. Bell RS, Mankin HJ, Doppelt SH. *J Bone Joint Surg* 1986;68A:1380-1388.

> Eleven of 49 patients followed by the authors had required admission to the hospital for an acute symptom complex. Five of the patients proved to have acute hematogenous osteomyelitis. Delayed diagnosis in three patients led to an unsatisfactory outcome. The authors suggest multiple blood cultures, bone scans, and either computed tomography or magnetic resonance imaging to help make an early diagnosis.

Fractures in children who have Gaucher's disease. Katz K, Cohen IJ, Ziv N, et al. *J Bone Joint Surg* 1987;69A:1361-1370.

> Three pathological fractures in nine children with Gaucher's disease are reported. Most fractures occurred between two and 12 months after a crisis. Fracture healing was prolonged. Inadequate periods of immobilization and early weightbearing led to malunion.

Tumors

Peter D. Pizzutillo, MD

Musculoskeletal Tumor Surgery. Enneking WF. New York, Churchill Livingstone, 1983.
> A detailed account of the surgical management of bone and soft-tissue tumors. Includes information on classification, description, and natural history.

Bone and soft tissue tumors. Springfield DS. In Morrissy RT (ed): *Pediatric Orthopaedics*. Philadelphia, JB Lippincott, 1990, pp 325-363.
> A well-written overview of the subject with emphasis on musculoskeletal tumors that occur in childhood.

Tumors and Tumorous Conditions of the Bones and Joints. Jaffe HL. Philadelphia, Lea & Febiger, 1979.
> A classic bone tumor pathology reference.

Evaluation and Diagnosis

Staging

A system for surgical staging of musculoskeletal sarcoma. Enneking WF, Spanier, SS, Goodman MA. *Clin Orthop* 1980;153:106-120
> The original reports on a staging system designed for both bone and soft-tissue tumors. Frequently used by orthopaedic surgeons, this system is especially useful for the surgeon planning treatment.

A system of staging musculoskeletal neoplasms. Enning WF. In Bassett FH III (ed): American Academy of Orthopaedic Surgeons *Instructional Course Lectures, XXXVII*. Park Ridge, IL, American Academy of Orthopaedic Surgeons, 1988, pp 3-10.
> The author describes the staging system for musculoskeletal neoplasms adopted by the Musculoskeletal Tumor Society and the American Joint Committee for Cancer Staging and End Results Reporting. Benign and malignant tumors are staged by categories of grade, site, and metastasis. Malignant tumors are classified as low grade or high grade based on histologic findings, radiographic assessment, and clinical correlation. The site or anatomic setting is either intracapsular, extracapsular but contained within the compartment, or extracapsular with extracompartmental extension. Metastases are either absent or present.

Metastasis to either regional nodes or distal sites has the same staging significance.

Treatment of the patient with stage MO soft tissue sarcoma. Suit H, Mankin HJ, Wood WC, et al. *J Clin Oncol* 1988;6:854-862.
> A revised staging system for soft-tissue sarcomas based on three histologic grades, three sizes, whether or not there is nodal involvement, and whether or not there is distant metastasis.

The evaluation of a soft-tissue mass in the extremities. Lange TA. In Barr JS Jr (ed): American Academy of Orthopaedic Surgeons *Instructional Course Lectures, XXXVIII.* Park Ridge, IL, American Academy of Orthopaedic Surgeons, 1989, pp 391-398.
Preoperative staging techniques for soft-tissue neoplasms. Makley JT. In Barr JS Jr (ed): American Academy of Orthopaedic Surgeons *Instructional Course Lectures, XXXVIII.* Park Ridge, IL, American Academy of Orthopaedic Surgeons, 1989, pp 399-405.
> These two recent review articles describe the thinking and decision-making in the preoperative evaluation of a soft-tissue mass in the extremities.

Magnetic Resonance Imaging and Computed Tomography

Magnetic resonance imaging of the musculoskeletal system in children. Hall TR, Kangarloo H. *Clin Orthop* 1989;244:119-130.
> A review of magnetic resonance imaging application in pediatrics with a good description of physiologic versus pathologic bone marrow changes.

Magnetic resonance imaging of primary tumours and tumour-like lesions of bone. Bohndorf K, Reiser M, Lochner B, et al. *Skeletal Radiol* 1986;15:511-517.
> Magnetic resonance imaging is a highly sensitive method for the detection of skeletal tumours. Plain films remain the most reliable method to assess biologic activity, grade, and probable histologic diagnosis.

Bone tumors: Magnetic resonance imaging versus computed tomography. Zimmer WD, Berquist TH, McLeod RA, et al. *Radiology* 1985;155:709-718.
> Magnetic resonance imaging is equal to or superior to computed tomography in demonstrating the extent of tumorous marrow and for delineating the extent of tumor in soft tissue. Computed tomography is superior for demonstrating calcific deposits and pathologic fractures. Magnetic resonance imaging is superior to computed tomography in documenting recurrent tumor because of artefactual degradation of the computed tomography image.

Pitfalls in the use of computed tomography for musculoskeletal tumors in children. Jones ET, Kuhns LR. *J Bone Joint Surg* 1981;63A;1297-1304.
> Computed tomography is a useful adjunct to the more conventional means of preoperative assesment, but overdependence on this one method of evaluation should be avoided.

Computed tomography of the musculoskeletal system Genant HK, Wilson JS, Bovill EG, et al. *J Bone Joint Surg* 1980;62A:1088-1101.
> The value for tumor management is in differentiating tumors from tumor-imitating lesions, demonstrating the extent of lesions, defining the relationship to adjacent neurovascular and other soft-tissue structures, revealing patterns of density, confirming metastatic lesions, resolving possible false positive results in radionuclide scanning, and evaluating recurrent disease.

Biopsy

Biopsy of musculoskeletal tumors. Simon MA. *J Bone Joint Surg* 1982;64A:1253-1257.
> A detailed description of biopsy techniques. Biopsy is to be used in association with a careful and complete diagnostic and staging sequence.

The hazards of biopsy in patients with malignant primary bone and soft-tissue tumors. Mankin HJ, Lange TA, Spanier SS. *J Bone Joint Surg* 1982;64A:1121-1127.
> Biopsy-related problems occurred from three to five times more frequently when the biopsy was performed at a referring institution rather than in a major treatment center.

Soft-Tissue Tumors

The management of soft-tissue sarcomas of the extremities. Simon MA, Enneking WF. *J Bone Joint Surg* 1976;58A:317-327.
> The location of the tumor and adequacy of the ablative surgery are the most important factors in determining the outcome of treatment.

The principles and technique of resection of soft parts for sarcoma. Bowden L, Booher RJ. *Surgery* 1958;44:963-977.
> Description of the surgical management of soft-tissue sarcomas based primarily on the anatomic site of the tumor. Amputation is performed when extensive resection of soft parts is not applicable.

Specific Lesions

Rhabdomyosarcoma in children and adolescents: A review. Ruymann FB. *Hematol Oncol Clin North Am* 1987;1:621-654.

Leiomyosarcomas in childhood: A clinical and pathologic study of ten cases. Lack EE. *Pediatr Pathol* 1986;6:181-197.

Malignant tumours in neonate. Campbell AN, Chan HS, O'Brien, et al. *Arch Dis Child* 1987;62:19-23.

Benign Bone Tumors

Benign Osteoblastoma

Osteoblastoma: Classification and report of 16 patients. Tonai M, Campbell CJ, Ahn GH, et al. *Clin Orthop* 1982;167:222-235.

> Cases are grouped as spinal, central benign, aggressive, and periosteal. The tumor can mimic aneurysmal bone cyst. Aggressive lesions can be distinguished on radiographic and histologic evidence. They must be differentiated from telangiectatic osteosarcoma. None became frankly malignant, but all required complete excision. The other lesions could be managed by marginal resection or curettage.

Benign osteoblastoma: Range of manifestations. Marsh BW, Bonfiglio M, Brady LP, et al. *J Bone Joint Surg* 1975;57A:1-9.

> The lesion has also been called osteogenic fibroma of bone and giant osteoid osteoma. The lesion exhibited a wide variation of biologic behavior. Clinical, roentgenographic, and histologic findings must be combined to distinguish the lesion from other closely related lesions such as osteoid osteoma and aneurysmal bone cyst. Treatment is discussed.

Benign osteoblastoma of the spine in childhood. Myles ST, MacRae ME. *J Neurosurg* 1988;68:884-888.

> Evaluates ten children with spinal osteoblastoma and gives the results of treatment. Excellent results were obtained with complete excision or partial excision of the osteoblastoma with bone grafting.

Osteoid Osteoma

Osteoid osteoma and osteoblastoma: Current concepts and recent advances. Healey JH, Ghelman B. *Clin Orthop* 1986;204:76-85.

> A review of the existing clinical knowledge as well as experience with imaging of the tumors and pathophysiology.

Osteoid-osteoma: Diagnostic problems. Sim FH, Dahlin DC, Beabout JW. *J Bone Joint Surg* 1975;57A:154-159.

> Fifty-four patients had the typical features of osteoid osteoma, but no histologic evidence of a nidus was found at initial surgery. Thirty-one were relieved of symptoms and required no further treatment. Three had

another diagnosis verified. A nidus was subsequently found at reoperation in nine. Five others became asymptomatic after reoperation even though no nidus was ever found.

Osteoid-osteoma as a cause of scoliosis. Keim HA, Reina EG. *J Bone Joint Surg* 1975;57A:159-163.

Nine cases of spinal osteoid osteoma caused a painful scoliosis. Almost all cases were misdiagnosed and improperly treated at first. Scoliosis was relieved by surgical excision of the lesion.

Osteoid osteoma and benign osteoblastoma of the spine: Clinical presentation and treatment. Kirwan EO, Hutton PA, Pozo JL, et al. *J Bone Joint Surg* 1984;66B:21-26.

Typical patient is a young person with pain, spinal stiffness, and scoliosis, which may become structural. Diagnosis is commonly delayed. Diagnostic and surgical management is discussed.

Scintigraphic patterns in osteoid osteoma and spondylolysis. Wells RG, Miller JH, Sty JR. *Clin Nucl Med* 1987;12:39:-44.

Osteoid osteoma and osteoblastoma of the spine in children: Report of 22 cases with brief literature review. Azouz EM, Kozlowski K, Marton D, et al. *Pediatr Radiol* 1986;16:25-31.

Osteoid osteoma of the proximal femur: New techniques in diagnosis and treatment. Kumar SF, Harcke HT, MacEwen GD, et al. *J Pediatr Orthop* 1984;4:669-672.

Precise localization of the lesion is accomplished by a combination of imaging techniques. Intraoperative localization and removal is aided by use of image intensifier and a sterile radiation probe. It is possible to remove a minimal amount of bone when resecting the lesion.

Negative radionuclide scan in osteoid osteoma: A case report. Fehring TK, Green NE. *Clin Orthop* 1984;185:245-249.

Case report of a patient, emphasizing that a negative bone scan does not preclude the diagnosis of osteoid osteoma. Multiple skeletal lesions in a 7-year-old girl.

Benign Cartilage Tumors

Benign and malignant cartilage tumors. Lewis MM, Sissons HA, Norman A, et al. In Griffin PP (ed): American Academy of Orthopaedic Surgeons *Instructional Course Lectures, XXXVI*. Park Ridge, IL, American Academy of Orthopaedic Surgeons, 1987, pp 87-114.

A good overview of the presentation, radiographic and pathologic findings, and treatment of benign and malignant cartilage tumors.

Osteochondroma

The origins of osteochondromas and endochondromas: A histopathologic study. Milgram JW. *Clin Orthop* 1983;174:264-284.
> Histopathologic sections from osteochondromas reveal aberrant cartilaginous epiphyseal growth-plate tissue that proliferates autonomously and separates from the normal growth plate at its edge.

Chondroblastoma

Chondroblastoma of bone: A critical review. Huvos AG, Marcove RC. *Clin Orthop* 1973;95:300-312.
> A review of this unusual tumor.

Benign chondroblastoma: A study of 125 cases. Dahlin DC, Ivins JC. *Cancer* 1972;30:401-413.
> Treatment recommended is en bloc resection, curettage with bone graft, or irradiation, depending on the accessibility of the tumor.

"Aggressive" chondroblastoma: Light and ultramicroscopic findings after en bloc resection. Mirra JM, Ulich TR, Eckardt JJ, et al. *Clin Orthop* 1983;178:276-284.
> Most chondroblastomas are relatively small lesions that respond favorably to curettage and packing with bone chips. In rare cases the lesions become very large; in others the lesions recur with or without soft-tissue seeding.

Chondromyxoid Fibroma

Chondromyxoid fibroma: The experience at the Istituto Ortopedico Rizzoli. Gherlinzoni F, Rock M, Picci P. *J Bone Joint Surg* 1983;65A:198-204.
> The presentation, incidence, and characteristics of chondromyxoid fibroma are described in this article with the success of the results of surgical treatment. The authors conclude that curettage combined with corticocancellous bone grafting is the treatment of choice for patients with chondromyxoid fibroma with significant decrease in recurrence rate.

Benign Tumors - Others

Aneurysmal Bone Cyst

Aneurysmal bone cyst after fracture: A report of three cases. Dabezies EJ, D'Ambrosia RD, Chuinard RG, et al. *J Bone Joint Surg* 1982;64A:617-621.
> A report of three cases of aneurysmal bone cyst developing after a fracture in the same area. Trauma is postulated to stimulate a reactive

process in normal bone, which results in an arteriovenous fistula in the involved bone. Also provides a review of current treatment concepts.

Aneurysmal bone cysts of the spine. Hay MC, Paterson D, Taylor TK. *J Bone Joint Surg* 1978;60B:406-411.
> Analysis of 14 new cases and 78 previously reported by other authors. Predilection noted for neural arch of lumbar spine. Treatment by total excision where possible.

Aneurysmal bone cyst: A pathological entity commonly mistaken for giant-cell tumor and occasionally for hemangioma and osteogenic sarcoma. Lichtenstein L. *Cancer* 1950;3:279-289.
> Classic. Also see Lichtenstein L: Aneurysmal bone cysts. Further observations. *Cancer* 1953;6:1228-1237.

Eosinophilic Granuloma

Eosinophil granuloma of the spine. Seimon LP. *J Pediatr Orthop* 1981;1:371-376.
> Six patients with seven lesions all healed spontaneously after conservative, symptomatic treatment. The author states that radiation therapy and surgical intervention should not be undertaken unless specific indications such as neurological complications warrant it.

Eosinophilic granuloma and its variations. Mickelson MR, Bonfiglio M. *Orthop Clin North Am* 1977;8:933-945.
> The characteristics and management of eosinophilic granuloma, Hand-Schuller-Christian disease, and Letterer-Siwe disease. They are also grouped by some authors as histiocytosis X.

Eosinophilic granuloma of bone. Makley JT, Carter JR. *Clin Orthop* 1986;204:37-44.

Fibrous Tumors of Bone

Bone tumors: Part II. Fibrous tumor of bone. Sim FH, Wold LE, Swee RG. In Murray JA (ed): American Academy of Orthopaedic Surgeons *Instructional Course Lectures, XXXIII.* St. Louis, CV Mosby, 1984, pp 40-59.
> Summarizes features and management for the following: Fibrous cortical defect (periosteal or cortical desmoid), metaphyseal fibrous defect (non-ossifying fibroma), desmoplasmic fibroma, congenital fibromatoses, fibrous dysplasia, and osteofibrous dysplasia.

Multiple skeletal fibroxanthomas: Radiologic-pathologic correlation of 72 cases. Moser RP Jr, Sweet DE, Haseman DB, et al. *Skeletal Radiol* 1987;16:353-359.

Fibrous dysplasia: An analysis of options for treatment. Stephenson RB, London MD, Hankin FM, et al. *J Bone Joint Surg* 1987;69A:400-409.

> This review of symptomatic lesions of fibrous dysplasia suggests satisfactory results of closed treatment of lesions of the upper extremity, but emphasizes the difficulty in treatment of lesions of the lower extremity even with surgical techniques. Internal fixation is frequently required in the lower extremity. Significant long-term morbidity is associated with this disease.

Unicameral Bone Cyst

Unicameral bone cyst (simple bone cyst). Makley JT, Joyce MJ. *Orthop Clin North Am* 1989;20:407-415.

> Review of the pathophysiology, activity, and treatment options for unicameral bone cyst.

Unicameral and aneurysmal bone cyst. Campanacci M, Capanna R, Picci P. *Clin Orthop* 1986;204:25-36.

Operative treatment versus steroid injection in the management of unicameral bone cysts. Oppenheim WL, Galleno H. *J Pediatr Orthop* 1984;4:1-7.

> A review of the characteristics and treatment of the lesion with a complete bibliography. Both surgical treatment and percutaneous steroid injection exhibited high rates of recurrence or persistence. The greater simplicity and less morbidity of steroid technique made it the method of choice.

Final results obtained in the treatment of bone cysts and methylprednisolone acetate (depo-medrol) and a discussion of results achieved in other bone lesions. Scaglietti O, Marchetti PG, Bartolozzi P. *Clin Orthop* 1982;165:33-42.

> Results in 163 simple bone cysts treated by injection. Also reports preliminary results for a small number of other benign bone lesions.

Giant Cell Tumors

Giant cell tumor of bone. Eckardt JJ, Grogan TJ. *Clin Orthop* 1986;204:45-58.

> Pathologic staging and surgical management based on accepted staging criteria are presented.

Giant-cell tumor of bone. Campanacci M, Baldini N, Boriani S, et al. *J Bone Joint Surg* 1987;69A:106-114.

> Gives the incidence, radiographic appearance, localization of tumor at presentation, and treatment of giant cell tumor in a population of 327 patients.

Giant-cell tumor of bone. McDonald DJ, Sim FH, McLeod RA, et al. *J Bone Joint Surg* 1986;68A:235-242.

>Mayo Clinic experience involving 221 patients with giant cell tumor is reported. Recurrence rate of 23% is noted most commonly in those undergoing curettage of the lesion. Curettage and bone grafts are the recommended treatments for most patients.

Giant-cell tumor of bone: An analysis of two hundred and eighteen cases. Goldenberg RR, Campbell CJ, Bonfiglio M. *J Bone Joint Surg* 1970;52A:619-664.

>An analysis of 218 cases of this uncommon tumor collected from multiple centers. Histologic findings of malignancy were important, but prognosis for recurrence or metastasis could not be based on benign histologic findings.

Malignant Bone Tumors

Chondrosarcoma

Chondrosarcoma in children and adolescents. Aprin H, Riseborough EJ, Hall JE. *Clin Orthop* 1982;166:226-232.

>Chondrosarcoma is rare in children. It has a relatively rapid onset manifested by pain, a palpable mass, and neurologic symptoms (if located in the spinal column). Treatment is by radical excision. Outcomes are poor in general, but better in lower grade lesions and in extremities, where adequate excision can be done.

Juxtacortical Chondrosarcoma

Periosteal chondrosarcoma and periosteal osteosarcoma: Two distinct entities. Bertoni F, Boriani S, Laus M, et al. *J Bone Joint Surg* 1982;64B:370-376.

>Review of 27 cases. Periosteal chondrosarcoma has a good prognosis and can even be treated by marginal excision in low-grade lesions. Periosteal osteosarcoma has a less satisfactory prognosis, but better than osteosarcoma. It can be treated by wide excision.

Ewing's Sarcoma and Other Round-Cell Tumors

Bone tumors: Part I. Small cell tumors of bone. Pritchard DJ. In Murray JA (ed): American Academy of Orthopaedic Surgeons *Instructional Course Lectures, XXXIII*. St. Louis, CV Mosby, 1984, pp 26-39.

>Ewing's sarcoma, lymphoma of bone, and neuroblastoma metastatic to bone. Summarizes clinical features, radiographic findings, laboratory findings, pathology findings, treatment, and prognosis.

Malignant bone tumor in children: Ewing's sarcoma. Meyers PA. *Hematol Oncol Clin North Am* 1987;1:667-673.

> Successful treatment of Ewing's sarcoma requires both radiation therapy and surgery for local control of primary tumors, as well as multi-agent protocols for chemotherapeutic control. Both radiation therapy and surgery have significantly better results when used in conjunction with effective chemotherapy.

Malignant Fibrous Histiocytoma

Malignant fibrous histiocytoma of soft tissue in childhood. Raney RB Jr, Allen A, O'Neill J, et al. *Cancer* 1986;57:2198-2201.

> Childhood malignant fibrous histiocytoma requires surgical removal for successful therapy; the role of chemotherapy and of radiation therapy are to be defined.

A clinicopathologic comparison of malignant fibrous histiocytoma and liposarcoma. Spanier SS, Floyd J. In Barr JS Jr (ed): American Academy of Orthopaedic Surgeons *Instructional Course Lectures, XXXVIII*. Park Ridge, IL, American Academy of Orthopaedic Surgeons, 1989, pp. 407-417

> The authors review in detail the histiologic features and clinical findings in 148 cases of malignant fibrous histiocytoma and 44 cases of liposarcoma. This is an excellent, up-to-date description of these two lesions.

Osteosarcoma

Magnetic resonance imaging of osteosarcomas: Comparison with computed tomography. Zimmer WD, Berquist TH, McLeod RA, et al. *Clin Orthop* 1986;208:289-299.

> Magnetic resonance imaging is equal to or superior to computed tomography for demonstrating tumor extent in marrow and for defining soft-tissue mass. Computed tomography is superior for demonstrating calcifications. Magnetic resonance imaging is of greatest value in the peripheral skeleton, in the medullary canal, and in soft tissue.

Adjuvant chemotherapy for osteosarcoma. Eilber FR, Rosen G. *Semin Oncol* 1989;16:312-323.

> Reviews the demographics, natural history, and historical perspective of chemotherapeutic treatment of osteosarcoma. Includes results of various combinations of chemotherapeutic agents and indicates advantages of preoperative use of chemotherapeutic agents.

Causes of increased survival of patients with osteosarcoma: Current controversies. Simon MA. *J Bone Joint Surg* 1984;66A:306-310.

> Surveys the improved results with modern treatment and analyzes the factors responsible. Extensive bibliography.

Pulmonary resection for metastatic osteogenic sarcoma. Spanos PK, Payne WS, Ivins JC, et al. *J Bone Joint Surg* 1976;58A:624-628.

> As a group, patients selected for lung resection had significantly longer survival than did patients whose pulmonary metastasis was untreated.

Skip metastases in osteosarcoma: Recent experience. Malawer MM, Dunham WK. *J Surg Oncol* 1983;22:236-245.

> Skip metastases are a grave prognostic sign despite adjuvant chemotherapy.

"Skip" metastases in osteosarcoma. Enneking WF, Kagan A. *Cancer* 1975;36:2192-2205

> Classic study of this finding, which occurred in 25% of their cases.

Osteosarcoma Variants

Osteosarcoma with small cells simulating Ewing's tumor. Sim FH, Unni KK, Beabout JW, et al. *J Bone Joint Surg* 1979;61A:207-215.

> Prognosis worse than osteosarcoma. Not radiosensitive.

Juxtacortical (parosteal) osteogenic sarcoma: Histological grading and prognosis. Ahuja SC, Villacin AB, Smith J, et al. *J Bone Joint Surg* 1977;59A:632-647.

> Good prognosis for grade I and grade II. Poor prognosis for grade III.

Periosteal osteogenic sarcoma. Unni KK, Dahlin DC, Beabout JW. *Cancer* 1976;37:2476-2485.

> Rare (1% of osteosarcomas seen at Mayo Clinic). Predominantly chondroblastic with fine lace-like osteoid trabeculae. Less prone to metastasis than conventional osteosarcoma.

Postradiation sarcoma of bone. Sim FH, Cupps RE, Dahlin DC, et al. *J Bone Joint Surg* 1972;54A:1479-1489.

> Malignant tumors were found in previously normal irradiated bones and in previously benign lesions treated by irradiation. The prognosis is poor.

Mimickers of Bone Tumors

Fracture callus associated with benign and malignant bone lesions and mimicking osteosarcoma. Kahn LB, Wood FW, Ackerman LV. *Am J Clin Pathol* 1969;52:14-24.

> Fracture callus superimposed on benign and malignant bone lesions may cause considerable diagnostic difficulty. Misinterpretation of this callus as osteosarcoma may lead to an unjustified amputation. The careful correlation of all available features of each case was found to be the most important factor in preventing errors.

Idiopathic cortical hyperostosis. Jones ET, Hensinger RN, Holt JF. *Clin Orthop* 1982;163:210-213.

> A benign condition that may be confused with bone tumors (especially osteoid osteoma, eosinophilic granuloma, and Ewing's sarcoma) or bone infections. This problem may be seen in older children, but usually occurs during infancy.

Rehabilitation

David P. Roye Jr, MD

Parent involvement in physical therapy: A controversial issue. Short DL, Schade JK, Herring JA. *J Pediatr Orthop* 1989;9:444-446.
> The authors emphasize the need to involve parents in the child's physical therapy. Parents in this study were able to reinforce formal physical therapy.

Severe orthopedic disability in childhood: Solutions provided by rehabilitation engineering. Bleck EE. *Orthop Clin North Am* 1978;9:509-528.
> Goal setting, seating, orthotics, and prosthetics are described for such individual disease entities as cerebral palsy and osteogenesis imperfecta congenita.

Ambulation

Energy cost of walking in normal children and in those with cerebral palsy: Comparison of heart rate and oxygen uptake. Rose J, Gamble JG, Medeiros J, et al. *J Pediatr Orthop* 1989;9:276-279.
> Makes interesting correlation between heart rate and oxygen consumption. Points out a simple way to evaluate and quantify results of rehabilitation and treatment.

Variations in the gait of normal children: A graph applicable to the documentation of abnormalities. Todd FN, Lamoreux LW, Skinner SR, et al. *J Bone Joint Surg* 1989;71A:196-204.
> Describes a method for evaluating gait dimensions in children, using only a stopwatch, in order to evaluate treatments and/or development. Describes the relationship between stride length, height, and walking speed.

Comparative assessment of gait after limb-salvage procedures. McClenaghan BA, Krajbich JI, Pirone AM, et al. *J Bone Joint Surg* 1989;71A:1178-1182.
> Demonstrates how oxygen consumption can be used to evaluate objectively the results of a reconstruction procedure.

Functional ambulation in patients with myelomeningocele. Hoffer MM, Feiwell E, Perry LR, et al. *J Bone Joint Surg* 1973;55A:137-148.
> A classic. Often used for other disabilities as well.

Limb Orthotics

Lower extremity orthotics. Engen TJ, Lehmkuhl LD. *Curr Orthop* 1989;3:194-200.
>Offers a comprehensive overview of lower extremity orthotic principles and application, with emphasis on the problems of paralysis of the lower extremity.

Clinical experience with the reciprocal gait orthosis in myelodysplasia. McCall RE, Schmidt WT. *J Pediatr Orthop* 1986;6:157-161.
>Reviews 41 patients treated with the reciprocal gait orthosis. Emphasizes the need to ambulate myelodysplasic patients.

A clinical review of the orthotic treatment of myelomeningocele patients. Rose GK, Sankarankutty M, Stallar J. *J Bone Joint Surg* 1983;65B:242-246.
>Demonstrates that functional ambulation is achievable in children with high levels of paralysis caused by myelomeningocele. Evaluates the use of the Salop skate, swivel walker, and hip guidance orthosis.

Current uses of mobility aids. Allison BJ. *Clin Orthop* 1980;148:62-69.
>Reviews the use of mobility aids ranging from parapodia to caster carts to motorized wheelchairs.

The "Gillette" sitting support orthosis. Carlson JM, Winter R. *Orthotics Prosthetics* 1978;32(4):35-45.
>A description of the fabrication and use of the Gillette sitting support orthosis.

Atlas of Orthotics: Biomechanical Principles and Application, ed 2. American Academy of Orthopaedic Surgeons. St. Louis, CV Mosby, 1985.
>This comprehensive reference source covers all aspects of current orthotic management. Includes relevant biomechanical sections and discussions of pathophysiology.

Lower extremity bracing: McCollough NC III: Part I. Introduction to lower extremity orthotics, pp 116-124. Fryer CM: Part II. Biomechanics of the lower extremity, pp 124-130. Lehneis HR: Part III. Principles of orthotic alignment in the lower extremity, pp 131-136. Glancy J: Part IV. Lower extremity orthotic components. Applications and indications, pp 136-154. In American Academy of Orthopaedic Surgeons *Instructional Course Lectures, XX*. St. Louis, CV Mosby, 1971.
>Comprehensive coverage of lower extremity bracing. Part I deals with rationale for bracing and analysis of the patient's need. Part II covers relevant biomechanics with kinetic and lower extremity function. Part III deals with orthotic adjustment. Part IV deals with practical applications and indications for orthotics.

Bracing for ambulation in childhood progressive muscular dystrophy. Spencer GE Jr, Vignos PJ Jr. *J Bone Joint Surg* 1962;44A:234-242.

Describes the usefulness of conventional orthotic management in prolonging ambulation in children with muscular dystrophy.

Recreation

Sports and recreational programs for the child and young adult with physical disability. Proceedings of the Winter Park Seminar. American Academy of Orthopaedic Surgeons, Winter Park, CO, April 11-13, 1983, pp 993-883.
A survey of programs available to the disabled child. Guidelines to assess participation possibilities for the individual child. Information for program development. Appendix references current athlete classification systems, literature, media, and other resources.

Brain Injury

Functional outcome of closed head injury in children and young adults. Eiben CF, Anderson TP, Lockman L, et al. *Arch Phys Med Rehabil* 1984;65:168-170.
Of 52 patients surveyed by questionnaire, 36 survivors included approximately 30% who were totally dependent, 30% who were partially dependent, and 40% who were independent. Younger patients with coma duration less than 21 days were more likely to be independent, but even after protracted coma, about a third became independent. Deficits in cognitive function and communication skills contributed proportionally more to disability than did problems in other areas.

Rehabilitation of brain injured children. Brink JD, Hoffer, MM. *Orthop Clin North Am* 1978;9:451-454.
Offers guidelines for predicting eventual prognosis and establishing realistic functional goals. Includes a brief discussion of early and later orthopaedic management.

Head Injuries. Hoffer M, Brink J, Marsh JS, et al. In Morrisey RT (ed): *Pediatric Orthopaedics*. Philadelphia, JB Lippincott, 1990, vol 2, pp 611-624.
Describes the evaluation, natural history, and orthopaedic (including surgical) management of children with head injuries.

Mental Retardation

The functional and social significance of orthopedics rehabilitation of mentally retarded patients with cerebral palsy. Hoffer MM, Bullock M. *Orthop Clin North Am* 1981;12:185-191.
Analyzes quality of life and cost of maintenance as a result of orthopaedic care.

Spinal Cord Injury

Spinal cord injury. Bonnet CA, Mitani M, Guess V. In Lovell WW, Winter RB (eds): *Pediatric Orthopaedics*. Philadelphia, JB Lippincott, 1978, vol 1, pp 495-531.

> Describes the medical and rehabilitation management of children with this injury.